# DOABLE

All Bible verses are from the King James Version of the Holy Bible, New International Version®, NIV®, Copyright©1973, 1978, 2011 by Biblica, Inc.® Used by permission. All rights reserved worldwide.

Copyright © 2020 by Cindy Leuty Jones
Published by Moraga Press
www.gocindyjones.com

Library of Congress Cataloging-in-Publication Data is available upon request.
ISBN: 978-1-7345676-0-1 (paperback)
ISBN: 978-1-7345676-1-8 (ebook)

Book design: Dania Zafar
Front cover graphic: Dimitrii Guzhanin/Shutterstock.com
Back cover photo: Nicole Bisek

First printing edition 2020.
Printed in the United States

# DOABLE

LITTLE DECISIONS THAT WILL
TRANSFORM YOUR LIFE

CINDY LEUTY JONES

To the love of my life, Jack.

I am because of him.

# CONTENTS

# Introduction

*What's so great about inspiration is sometimes*
*it finds you when you're not looking.*
—WONG KAR-WAL, FILM DIRECTOR

YOU baby! This book is the definitive guide to creating the best YOU and the best life for YOU. Yeah, baby! It's all about YOU.

The first time I tried to make pancakes, it didn't go so well. The skillet may have been too hot, the batter too thick, too thin—whatever. The skillet was smoking with misshapen burnt dough blobs. I threw the whole thing out and started over.

We make mistakes. Some are temporary setbacks—like burnt pancakes. Some we chalk up as a lesson learned, like how not to burn the pancakes. Others might be epic fails with disastrous consequences, like accidentally setting the kitchen on fire because you threw the smoldering pancakes into the trash.

As with my pancake adventure, trying anything new opens the doors for mistakes. Often, the first time we do anything, it doesn't go exactly as planned. Maybe we're able to rethink our process and try another way. Sometimes we get frustrated and chuck the whole mess. The first time trying something new can be a trial-and-error process of discovery and experimentation, or more like randomly throwing darts and hoping for the best.

Inevitably, mistakes are part of being human.

**The only man who never makes a mistake
is the man who never does anything.**
−THEODORE ROOSEVELT

Mistakes are defined as actions or judgments that are misguided or wrong. A mistake can also be an error in our action, a miscalculation, or the result of poor reasoning, carelessness, insufficient knowledge—must I go on? We mess up. We look back, find ways we might have circumvented our mistakes and limited or avoided the negative consequences.

We tell ourselves that next time we'll be smarter—but will we?

It takes a lot of effort to learn from our mistakes. You'd think we would make every effort not to make another mistake. But we move too fast, don't evaluate the options, think we know what we are doing, and convince ourselves that we've got it all figured out when many times we're far from having anything figured out. Our brain is lazy and wants to automate as much as possible, even if it's wrong. Mistakes, pitfalls, and mishaps—we're so prone to making them, it's a wonder any of us make it through life at all.

Screw up once and it's a mistake. Keep repeating the mistake and it becomes your decision. Conscious or unconscious, repeated mistakes become our decisions and decisions become our habits. Left unchecked, over a lifetime, bad habits can have negative consequences for the trajectory of our lives.

**Insanity: Doing the same things over and over
again and expecting different results.**
−UNKNOWN

*Doable* lays out the reasons why we make so many mistakes and how to avoid them. Delving into the neurological process of our shortcomings, we can explore and change the patterns holding us back. Then build new neural pathways to create your best life ever. This book will give you a road map to rethinking the choices you make, from your most basic physiological needs, to love, to your intellectual pursuits, and more. The goal is to be a fully-developed, self-actualized human being living the life meant for you.

It's estimated the average adult makes a whopping 35,000 remotely conscious decisions every day, with about 225 on food alone, according to researchers at Cornell University.[1] My guess is, for most of these little daily decisions, we could do better.

It's all about the little decisions that lead to big outcomes. When you take the daily little decisions for granted, the big picture can get lost. The long-term impact of your little decisions can create a life filled with vision and purpose. You're the accumulation of what you do every day, and that's a good thing because you can change your life right now by simply changing the little things.

Your life is the result of all your little decisions.

> **When you wake up every day, it's like a new birthday: it's a new chance to be great again and make great decisions.**
> —POO BEAR, AMERICAN RECORDING ARTIST

The phrase "the devil's in the details" has to do with making mistakes that sometimes snowball into epic failures. Maybe you forgot a step, thought a shortcut would work, or unconsciously made an innocent mistake. Everything after that chain reacted into one colossal screwup, causing you to back up, completely start over, or give up altogether.

Then there is the opposite phrase, "God is in the details," meaning that attention paid to the smallness will make the largeness possible. Digging into the details creates an opportunity for discovery and creativity, sparking our deepest curiosity to figure things out.

The same is true with our behaviors and habits. When we understand the reasons behind our actions, we rethink and make the best-choice outcomes for our lives.

Do you wonder what drives you?

We look at the social narrative, listen to the advice of others like parents and friends, and try to figure out what box we fit in. If we choose poorly, the box becomes a trap. Instead, how about breaking out of the box and being open to unlimited opportunities?

> *The secret of concentration is the secret of self-discovery. You reach inside yourself to discover your personal resources, and what it takes to match them to the challenge.*
> —ARNOLD PALMER, AMERICAN PROFESSIONAL GOLFER

## WHY I WROTE THIS BOOK

There's usually a reason why we set off on a path of self-discovery and self-improvement. Sometimes life just didn't go as planned and we stop to reevaluate. The process of learning more about ourselves often gets triggered by some life event—therapy, divorce, graduating from college, changing career paths, or we just wake up and decide today is the day to make some changes. The fact you're reading this book shows you're ready to discover something new about yourself.

For me, it was lying on a couch for a year that made me ask myself, "Why am I here?"

# LIFE-CHALLENGING EVENT NUMBER ONE

Through adversity, one grows and rethinks the trajectory of one's life.

Well, I've had a few redirects that have caused me to rethink, reevaluate, and reboot my operating system. We walk on the edge of a knife and could fall off either way, sometimes into the abyss of chaos and uncertainty, or to the side of clarity and a sense of purpose. I've been on both sides—a few times.

In 2008, I spent the entire year on the couch, sucking down several rounds of antibiotics. I didn't know it at the time, but my sinus cavities had closed off and were infected so badly that the infection occasionally seeped into the meninges of my brain.

Picture the worst flu you have ever had with a migraine and a tequila hangover, and quadruple it. It was a miserable time for me.

I spent that year watching a lot of movies, too brain-dead to read, meandering aimlessly around the house, and feeling beaten down. I was weak. I had no stamina, and my muscle tone was shriveling away. Even with all that, I noticed something I had never experienced before: my joints ached with searing pain.

I can't overstate how difficult this time was for me. It wasn't only the physical toll but the emotional toll. It takes a lot to be sick. Your life is on hold. Your patience is stretched. Time—takes—forever—to—pass. I wondered, If this is living, is it worth it? Do I need to be here?

Before my illness, I had been a pretty good athlete. I regularly did yoga and was an avid hiker. That's why it was so shocking. Constantly feeling lousy with aching, burning joints, fatigue, and flu-like symptoms had become my new normal. I wondered, Is it age? Arthritis? Being sick? Diet? What is going on?

During this time, while lying on the couch, I saw several news blurbs about Dara Torres. She was a forty-one-year-old mother who was setting off to accomplish what no other Olympian had ever done: competing in her fifth Olympics. She was the only woman in history to swim in the Olympics after the age of forty.[2]

In the lead-up to the Olympics, magazines and TV shows featured her in the gym doing some very impressive maneuvers with massive weights. She was focused, determined, and razor-sharp. It got my attention. I perked up and wondered, Why her and not me? Is it genetics? Training? Sheer determination? What gives? I needed to know.

After a scan of my sinuses, the determination was I needed surgery to reopen closed passageways that were causing my repeated infections. After the obligatory month of recovery, I went to the gym and hired a personal trainer. I decided to do what I could and see where it took me—maybe not to the Olympics, but at least off the couch.

I started to build my strength up again. Stand-up paddleboarding was beginning to catch on, so I tried it out. Paddleboarding is a water sport where you stand on an oversized, thick surfboard and have a canoe-like paddle that you use to heave-ho stroke your way through the ocean. I liked it, and over the next year of practice I got pretty darn good at it.

📌

It's really hard to conquer the world when you feel lousy.

I decided to enter a local paddleboard race. In a competition, you go a certain distance, maneuver around buoys, and make your way back to a finish line. In my first ocean race, there were about twenty competitors. I was the only woman and the oldest. I came in twelfth. I felt great! I was off the couch into a lifestyle of fitness and health.

And feeling great is what it's all about—feeling great about yourself, physically, emotionally, and mentally.

It's not easy lying on a couch for a year. Putting the apocalyptic health scare I faced behind me, I took the time to get my strength back, train, and focus on my body's health and well-being.

All this led me to wonder about every facet of my life—love, creativity, finances, where I lived, what car I drove, cat or dog—definitely dog. I wanted to take the opportunity to rebuild a life full of solid choices and productive habits, but I was overwhelmed with where to start—with what should come first in the chicken-or-egg thinking process.

I knew I needed a road map. I checked out all the self-help books, but nothing was hitting the aha in me.

The illness forced me to put my body's recovery first. As with any illness, you feel so terrible that critical thinking and emotional feeling aren't even on your radar. During my illness, I was so downcast I couldn't have cared less or felt less motivated about anything. Everything gets put on hold. I concluded, if the body is unwell, then the brain doesn't have a chance. The body must come first for the brain to flourish.

### *The chief function of the body is to carry the brain around.*
—THOMAS EDISON

Like the lyrics of a song stuck in my head, Thomas Edison's quote kept replaying in my brain. The body must come first, as the body is the portal for the brain's actions. The body provides the brain with a way to speak, share ideas, hear, converse, see, touch, create, dance, smell flowers, feel the ocean water, and experience all the other wonders of the human body.

The body is the brain's home.

**_Take care of your body. It's the only place you have to live._**
—JIM BROWN, AMERICAN ENTREPRENEUR

Self-discovery is exploring and understanding your character and purpose in life. Along the way, there's a lot to ponder, values to sort out, and decisions to make. I've thought long and hard about this, and I find three things matter most in life: the health of your body, love in all its forms, and knowledge to help you discover your purpose in life.

For us to even exist, our fragile bodies must be protected, fed, and nourished. Everything starts with our health. We reside in our physical, material world—you can see, hear, smell, and touch. We can also be seen, heard, smelled, and touched by other people, or in prehistoric times by predators, like a saber-tooth tiger, who would like nothing better than to eat us. The material world is your body and everything within and around it. It's physical life itself.

In our brain, our consciousness, we swing between emotional feelings—the need for love—and intellectual reasoning—the need for purpose. But we are not binary, It's not an either or but a combination of both. We crave to have our emotional needs fulfilled, and when it comes to love, we need loads of it—from romantic partners, family, community, and other groups. We thrive when we are connected to others.

Our intellectual pursuits reward us with a sense of accomplishment and a sense of purpose. Accomplishments are a direct result of satisfying our sense of curiosity, learning new skills, and nurturing our intellectual pursuits to help us figure out what we're meant to do with our life.

Our consciousness, unlike our body, is not in our physical, material world. It's somewhere floating around in the weirdness of our brain where strings of chemicals spark neurons that somehow magically let us know chocolate is delicious. Our consciousness tells us how to spell a word, comprehend a mathematical equation, or feel an immediate, deep love for our newborn child. The consciousness, awareness, soul, mind, brain, spirit, essence, or whatever you want to call all those syntactical connections going on in our head is what makes us who we are. When it comes to our consciousness, so much has been discovered but it's considered a drop in the bucket of what is yet to come.

*Consciousness is a fascinating but elusive phenomenon ...*
*Nothing worth reading has been written on it.*
—STUART SUTHERLAND, BRITISH PSYCHOLOGIST

These three things—life, love, and purpose—define who you are and how you choose to live your life. The moments in your life that define you most are not scheduled on a calendar but happen based on the choices you make along the way.

*Watch your thoughts for they become words,*
*watch your words for they become actions,*
*watch your actions, for they become habits,*
*watch your habits for they become your character,*
*watch your character for it becomes your destiny.*
—RALPH WALDO EMERSON, AMERICAN ESSAYIST

# LIFE

Life is about our body, every cell, and how it all functions. It's also about the environment around us that affects the well-being of our bodies. We wouldn't live long unless we had shelter that protected us from the harsh environment, and we also need protection from things that could harm us. Whether it was a prehistoric wooly mammoth coming at us or a car dangerously swerving into our lane on the freeway—we need safety from things that can kill us.

Our body functions need air, water, food, sleep, and sex. The littlest thing can make a big difference. You'll discover the science behind how better posture can lead to significantly more oxygen to fire your brain. Drinking water as soon as you wake up can be more vital than that cup of coffee. The food you eat can be either the safest, most potent form of medicine or the slowest form of poison.

We deal with our environment through our fight-or-flight mode that can hijack our senses, creating unwarranted anxiety over things unlikely to harm us. We have the same fight-or-flight response, whether it's a saber-tooth tiger coming at us or our tax deadline fast approaching.

Life is concerned with every aspect of our material world.

> **To keep the body in good health is a duty ... otherwise,**
> **we shall not be able to keep our mind strong and clear.**
> —BUDDHA

# LOVE

Love conquers all. Feelings of love have been proven to thwart the negative emotions of fear, anger, anxiety and even stress. And the best place for love is to start with you. Before all else, you must love yourself first. Loving yourself opens you to see the love in others.

We also need to feel accepted, to be part of a family, community or our tribe. This belonging is so vital to our well-being that research has shown loneliness can prolong illness and increase your risk of dying prematurely. Our need for acceptance is a key ingredient to our very survival and happiness.

We may also long for romance and that special someone to share our life. Later in the book, I'll give you two dealbreaker questions to ask yourself before you tie your life and future to that special person.

*Only a life lived for others is a life worth living.*

—ALBERT EINSTEIN

# PURPOSE

Your purpose in life is the reason you get up in the morning. Purpose can influence behavior, shape our goals, create meaning in our lives and guide our life's direction. Purpose makes our work meaningful and satisfying, knowing we are contributing to ourselves, our families and to society as a whole.

Our curiosity entices us to learn and acquire a bank of knowledge. What you learn sets you on a path to discover how you can use your knowledge and talents to develop your ultimate purpose in life. But purpose can be found in everything we do; from learning a new recipe for dinner to making ground-braking scientific advances. Great or small, everything we do can have a deeper more meaningful purpose. A new recipe offers a new creative way to supply nutrients to ourselves and our family, ground-breaking scientific advances could better everyone's life.

Fulfilling our sense of curiosity is like breathing air for the intellect: our intellect won't flourish without it. Our curiosity has helped us to survive by creating new and better tools, skills, languages, arts and other things. It's enabled us to continually change, adapt, and find new and creative ways to live. Our sense of purpose is as individual as our very being, from discovering new scientific advances that change the world to new recipes for dinner. Curiosity and awe will lead you to wonder, to ask questions, to learn, and will guide you to discover how to fill your life with purpose, both great and small.

*I have no special talents. I am only passionately curious.*

—ALBERT EINSTEIN

I don't have all the answers, but I have the questions. The questions to ask yourself about your decisions, which lead to your life choices and create your future. There's no one-size-fits-all, and only you have the answers that are best for you.

**Alice: *"I just wanted to ask you which way I ought to go."***

**Cheshire Cat: *"Well, that depends on where you want to get to."***

**Alice: *"Oh, it really doesn't matter, as long as I—."***

**Cheshire Cat: *"Then it really doesn't matter which way you go."***

—ALICE IN WONDERLAND

One is not whole without the other; the body-mind connection is a two-way street.

Our emotions, how we think and feel, are so connected to how we feel physically. If you're depressed, your work suffers. Or if you're exhausted, children playing become annoying instead of joyful. If your body is unwell, then the function of the brain usually doesn't have a chance. And put that thought in reverse: if the brain is not making good choices, the body also suffers.

The brain to the body and the body to the brain—it's a two-way street.

If you let poor eating habits and a sedentary lifestyle be your mindless habit, heart disease, diabetes, or a stroke may become a life-threatening roadblock in your life. If your brain is prone to unchecked anger, anxiety, and stress, then your body will house that damage like a ticking time bomb. Statistics show people with high levels of anger, anxiety, and stress may also be more likely to have heart disease, diabetes, and stroke in their future. Honestly, if the body goes, there goes life itself.

> **If I knew I was going to live this long,**
> **I'd have taken better care of myself.**
> —MICKEY MANTLE, BASEBALL PLAYER

The brain and the body are connected. You've heard this before, but has it sunk in? In this book, you'll discover the intricacies of what it truly means. In turn, you'll use what you learn to your advantage and create your own remarkable life.

## CHAPTER ONE

# Habits, Mindlessness, and Autopilot

*All human actions have one or more of these*
*seven causes: chance, nature, compulsions,*
*habit, reason, passion, desire.*

— ARISTOTLE

Habits are a series of little decisions all connected that make up our daily routines. But how are they formed, and how do you start changing the ones that don't serve your awesomeness?

There are all kinds of habits: good, bad, endearing, annoying, nervous, healthy, unhealthy—and we, as humans, are defined as creatures of habit. Habits are something we often do, a pattern of action, a tendency to behave in a certain way.

*Nothing so needs reforming as other people's habits.*

—MARK TWAIN

A *Psychology Today* headline reads, "New Study Shows Humans Are on Autopilot Nearly Half the Time." Meaning we move somewhat rudderless through the routine of the day, as much of our daily life consists of the habits that we've formed. If half the actions of our day are driven by habits, then why is it so hard to build new and useful ones? It comes down to the difference between habitual mindlessness versus the intentional decisive mind.[3] Or, in other words, awareness.

In an experiment on mindless eating, participants tasted fresh and stale popcorn, and (as expected) they preferred the taste of fresh popcorn. When participants were offered popcorn at a movie theater, people ate just as much whether their popcorn was stale or fresh. The habit of combining the moviegoing experience with eating popcorn was so strong; it didn't matter if the popcorn was stale. The mindless habit won out.[4]

When it comes to bad habits, it all would be so much easier if we never developed bad habits in the first place. If we never picked up a cigarette, ate fast food, drank too much alcohol, missed restorative sleep, swore, bit our fingernails, drank too much coffee, binge-watched TV, racked up credit card debt, checked social media every five minutes, ate sugary treats, and whatever else comes to mind, but in some of those cases— we did. And therein lies the problem. Our bad habits don't propel us forward but tether us to repeating mistakes.

> **Tis easier to prevent bad habits than to break them.**
> —BENJAMIN FRANKLIN

## REPEAT PERFORMANCE

We've been told making a mistake can be a "learning experience." We did something wrong, made a mistake, and then used that mistake as a lesson learned.

Unfortunately, research indicates it's much harder to avoid repeating mistakes than we think. For better or worse, everything you do creates embedded neural pathways that become like roadways for your decisions and habits. We're more likely to repeat the actions because, by default, we slip back into the existing neural pathways that were created for whatever situation we're facing. Your neural pathways, like well-traveled roadways, are familiar paths of travel and easily repeatable.

Ruminating over your mistakes might even cause you to reopen that neural pathway for yet another trip down memory lane and to repeat the exact same mistake. Dwelling opens the door again for an encore performance. Our brains do learn from our mistakes—the problem is the brain learns how to continue making them, sometimes over and over and over.

In times of stress, when we're angry or filled with worry, we tend to throw gasoline on the fire by ruminating over other unrelated stresses and past poor choices, all adding to feelings of self-doubt. To alleviate the stress of the situation, we may revert to previous poor behaviors, especially if something about the behavior was pleasurable.

Our established neural pathways feel familiar and comforting regardless of whether they lead to positive or negative behaviors. The fact we've done them before is what's comforting. The neural pathway forms a habit loop. A negative self-belief triggers a pleasurable but poor behavior to alleviate the stress. Then, we feel ashamed for our poor behavior and feel the negative self-belief is justified. Then the loop repeats.

For example, maybe you messed up and are feeling bad about yourself. Adding to that, you start ruminating over all your past mistakes and feelings of failure and self-doubt arise. To alleviate the negative feelings, you decide to have a few drinks with friends. A few drinks wind up with you getting drunk. Even though you know getting drunk is a bad choice, you still drank too much anyway. Now, you feel your negative self-beliefs are justified because you got drunk. The loop repeats.

Self-destructive behaviors like being attracted to the wrong kind of person, using drugs to alleviate negative thoughts, binge-eating to relieve stress, or overspending to reward yourself are easy patterns to fall into, and tough to break.

Here's the secret: maybe it's better not to think backward at our past mistakes or let yourself ruminate over what's happened. I know it sounds simple, but think about how many times you have been down on yourself for a mistake. What would it have looked like if you had turned that around? If instead, you looked forward to what you wanted to accomplish and who you wanted to be in life.

Not dwelling on your mistakes takes the negative power out of it. It's great if you can learn from the bad, but it's even better to focus on the good you want to come into your life.

Instead of mindlessly lapsing into negative habits, develop a new strategy to handle trigger situations. Learn solutions that build positive neural pathways that you happily reinforce now and for your awesome future. Start to recognize thoughts or actions that don't serve you and instead choose ones that do.

Let the energy of future good decisions propel you in the direction you choose to create. Your thoughts are your choice. Learn to recognize thoughts and patterns that are harmful and hold you back.

***Smart people learn from their mistakes.***
***But the real sharp ones learn from the mistakes of others.***
—BRANDON MULL, AMERICAN AUTHOR OF CHILDREN'S BOOKS

## HABITS AND UNCERTAINTY

Since habits are such a massive part of your day, bad habits can trip you up and derail your life like nothing else. They're hard to break. It takes effort, focus, and determination. Editing bad habits from your life and embedding good habits are two skills that can lead you to a pretty awesome life. It's as simple as that—but saying and doing are worlds apart.

The good news is habits—all habits, good and bad—are learned behaviors. Just as you learned to ride a bike, operate a cell phone, or cook an egg, you can also learn more productive, useful habits.

Developing good habits means developing awareness and a focus on change. It takes a conscious effort, but good habits can be developed and maintained. Just like the bad habits, any good habit, over time, can successfully be integrated into a relaxed and comfortable part of your routine and become your new automated mindlessness. And that's the goal, to have your autopilot be on course to live your best life possible.

> **A nail is driven out by another nail:**
> **habit is overcome by habit.**
> —ERASMUS, DUTCH PHILOSOPHER

Habits are routines we've fallen into that can be defined by a three-part loop: A trigger or cue, followed by your response, which then evokes a reward.

It's the loop of a cue, a response, and then a reward that spins us into the mindless rinse and repeat of all good and bad habits that can loop over and over. Because the cues that cause habits, and how to change them are somewhat unique to each individual, there are entire books written on the subject. *Atomic Habits* by James Clear and *How Habits Work* by Charles Duhigg are two excellent books that go into detail on the deconstruction of habits, and how to create habits that benefit your life.

For my purposes, I have a slightly different take—baby steps before running.

The triggers, cravings, responses, routines, and rewards occur with all habits. There's no getting around that—but what if we wiped the slate clean and started at zero? What habits or life would we build? What cues or desires would we embed? Would putting the power of little decisions into play help the big decisions craft themselves? In this book, we'll do just that. We'll call out our daily, mindless decisions in order to craft the big decisions that will power our life.

In the next chapter, you'll discover the science and purpose behind these daily decisions that can change your life. But first, here's more of my take on habits.

Let's say your favorite coffee shop started offering freshly baked pastries right next to the cashier. The cue: a Danish pastry fresh from the oven. Your craving and response is to buy the yummy pastry. The reward? It's a Danish pastry, it's freaking delicious, and your brain lights up like sugar plum fairies with every bite. This becomes your morning ritual, and after several weeks of your daily pastry indulgence, your pants are hard to button up and way too tight to sit comfortably.

Simply put, a habit formed.
You saw it.
You liked it.
You wanted it.
You got it.

The problem is it all became routine, mindless behavior that eventually leads to a negative impact on your life. Now, your options are to spend money to buy new larger-sized pants or restrict your calories to lose weight. Neither option sounds like fun nor benefits your life. No one wants to spend money on pants you already own, and no one wants to be on a diet.

Our habits are comforting because they're predictable—even the bad ones. One of our greatest fears is the fear of the unknown or uncertainty. Our brains evolved memory to be able to predict things. Our early ancestors most likely felt safer when they knew what was coming. They probably memorized their migration patterns, what was over the next horizon, or where they could find food. This predictability would have aided in their very survival, and that truth is embedded in our brain.

We still crave predictability. In today's world, many of us are more likely to talk to someone we have spoken to before, even if they're downright dull as dirt, instead of venturing out of our comfort zone to talk to someone new. The certainty of a mediocre experience can be more comforting than the uncertainty and fear of putting yourself out there to talk to a new person—the unknown.

With bad habits comes familiarity, and if we're looking to decrease our uncertainty, a bad habit is comforting, even if it is not to our advantage. Uncertainty can be painful, and our bodies respond negatively to it, both physically and mentally. When our routine is altered, we may feel stymied. Our brain is frazzled, and we go from fear to possibly anger and frustration. The brain can become defiant when challenged.

Changing bad habits can be downright uncomfortable. So uncomfortable, there needs to be a smaller, baby step. If you want to move from A to B, the first step from A is not to leap directly to B, but to go from A to not doing A. First, you must let go of your routine and step into the fear of change—the very place we try to avoid, into the unknown. The unknown of how we can deal with the fear of uncertainty, even in the slightest way, like not ordering the Danish pastry today.

Tomorrow is another day. It takes one shovel-full of dirt at a time when trying to dig yourself out of the hole of bad habits. It's enough to know you can live with the uncomfortable and get through it. Let your first step be letting go of the behavior by "not doing A." Let it be getting comfortable with the undoing of the negative behavior. Be open to uncertainty and be open to learning something new. To learn something new, you have to risk. You have to let go.

*Your net worth to the world is usually determined by what remains after your bad habits are subtracted from your good ones.*
—BENJAMIN FRANKLIN

## WANT AND WILL

There's a difference between want and will. When someone wants something—it's a desire that may or may not be in the future, like wanting to buy a house. *Want* doesn't lead to a solid plan but conveys more an attitude. Everyone wants, but to have the *will* is where you step on the gas and put a plan in place.

*Will* means to express an action that you intend to do or perform, like saying you will buy a house. Will is a commitment to your future. It's more concrete.

*What does it take to be a champion? Desire, dedication, determination, concentration, and the will to win.*
—PATTY BERG, PROFESSIONAL GOLFER

## ARE YOU IN 100 PERCENT?

As we've discussed, habits are behaviors that are repeated over and over again until they reach an unconscious repetition in our lives. Labeling habits as good or bad empowers them with emotions that may not serve you well. Instead, relabel them and use *healthy* or *unhealthy* or maybe *empowering* or *not empowering*. This little step will shift the dynamic.

Healthy habits are ones that empower you and help make your life better.

Unhealthy habits are ones that are detrimental to your future, slowing or reversing the progress and trajectory of your life.

Habits are hard enough to change without imbuing them with emotions that don't serve you. Our unhealthy habits can be comforting as a way to avoid stress, or they may arise out of convenience. Eating fast food daily is an example of a convenient and unhealthy habit. Smoking is an example of an unhealthy habit that is used to reduce stress.

We know we also fear change. Change is uncomfortable. Change takes work and commitment to yourself.

The key is to be 100 percent open to change.

Say what?

Yep, it's all about being present 100 percent, being committed 100 percent, and taking responsibility 100 percent. That may sound like a lot, but studies show being 100 percent committed is easier than being "kind of" committed.

For example, when getting married, how would you feel if instead of saying, "I do," your future spouse said, "Yeah, I'll give it a shot." Being 100 percent is when the decision has been made, and you burn the ship behind you—no escape routes. You move forward. When you're this committed, results happen.

Believe you can do it. With attention and focus, you can do anything. You have to believe in yourself and love yourself.

Loving yourself will give you power. Are you ready to go the distance? 100 percent?

*Until one is committed, there is hesitancy, the chance to draw back, always ineffectiveness. Concerning all acts of initiative (and creation), there is one elementary truth, the ignorance of which kills countless ideas and splendid plans: that the moment one definitely commits oneself, then Providence moves too. All sorts of things occur to help one that would never otherwise have occurred. A whole stream of events issues from the decision, raising in one's favour all manner of unforeseen incidents and meetings and material assistance, which no man could have dreamt would have come his way. I have learned a deep respect for one of Goethe's couplets: Whatever you can do, or dream you can, begin it. Boldness has genius, power, and magic in it!*

—WILLIAM HUTCHISON MURRAY, SCOTTISH MOUNTAIN CLIMBER

## BACK TO ME

Okay, after several months of personal training sessions, I did start to build some new muscles—but it wasn't easy.

When I woke up on training days, my brain started a negative conversation with me. Trying to find valid reasons to cancel, I kvetched about the pain in my neck: I must have slept wrong, and maybe I should cancel my session? My stomach was a little upset, and perhaps I should cancel? I'm sore, and maybe I should cancel? The sky is blue, so ... maybe I should cancel my session? I found myself dreaming up more and more creative ways to cancel. Like an out-of-control puppy first put on a leash, I resisted.

It was clear: I was my own worst enemy.

Going from point A—being out of shape, to point B—being fit—was too big a leap for my brain to comprehend. It's scary for the brain to think so far ahead and make lofty goals. The pressure sets in. It can be frightening and frustrating: since daily, incremental progress is hard to see, we then might only see ourselves not reaching our goal. I needed smaller doable steps so I could get comfortable with the process and not just focused on the goal.

I broke it down. I had to go from A to not A in the littlest way. The first step from point A to point B was to let go of A. I had to let go of being out of shape. Then I could take the first step without having the pressure of future expectations.

I made one decision: that I was not going to be the out-of-shape person I was.

I soon realized that on those days I did get up and go, and did what I could, like a miracle elixir, I always felt better. Even on the days I did an easy, no-sweat workout, I left the gym with an uplifted outlook and feeling refreshed.

That pushed me to make a deal with myself. No matter what, I would go. If, after ten minutes, I didn't want to be there, I could leave and do something else I enjoyed, but I had to show up. Nike's motto, Just Do It, was my mantra, but with a little twist: Just Show Up.

### *Eighty percent of success is showing up.*
—WOODY ALLEN

Months later, my workout sessions miraculously started to show results. People commented on my arms looking buff, that I looked fit, and seemed more upbeat. I heard comments about how I must love to workout. Let me be clear: I don't love working out. It is hard. But I decided to take the emotions out of it and not love it or hate it. I just let it be something I did. I put it in the same category as flossing my teeth. Most people don't love or hate flossing their teeth; they just do it. Going to the gym became my new mindless habit. To show up and see where the training session took me. No expectations. No negative conversations. I put it on my schedule and took it out of my emotions.

This one act of stopping the useless chatter in my head and being 100 percent committed to just showing up led me to build a much stronger body and a stronger mind.

Recovering from my illness and building up my strength may have been my motivation, but it took the habit and 100 percent commitment to get me out of the hole.

## WHAT NEXT?

Now that the body was working pretty well, I wondered, what else could I revamp in my life? Where would I begin? What comes next?

After the illness and now spectacular recovery, I realized anything was doable. The pressure was on: This is my life, and how do I want to live the rest of it?

The little decisions got my body back. So what else? I needed a road map of all the other little decisions that could change my life for the better.

*Motivation is what gets you started.*
*Habit is what keeps you going.*
—JIM RYUN, AMERICAN TRACK AND FIELD ATHLETE

**CHAPTER SUMMARY**

☑ There's no small decision or small habit.

☑ Creating habit only comes through deep concentration and daily consistency until your habits become a new positive lifestyle.

☑ Never let temporary failure be an excuse to give up.

☑ Thank you, Nike. I just did it. I showed up and did it. I just showed up and ventured into the unknown.

## CHAPTER TWO

# Me and Maslow

*The hallmark of successful people is that they are*
*always stretching themselves to learn new things.*
—CAROL S. DWECK, PROFESSOR OF PSYCHOLOGY AT STANFORD UNIVERSITY

To start creating positive daily habits, I looked at successful people to see how they organized their lives. What habits did they prioritize? What worked for them? I still needed a road map to organize the multitude of practices every life has into productive choices.

Successful people are just ordinary people with extraordinary habits.

I remembered Abraham Maslow and his famed theory about the hierarchy of needs as the motivation for all our behaviors. My motivation was to feel good. I wondered where that fit in his hierarchy of needs. It led me to rediscover Abraham Maslow, and his "road map" that might be the help I needed.

Abraham Maslow was an American psychologist best known for his hierarchy of needs theory from his paper "A Theory of Human Motivation," published in 1943, in *Psychological Review* and later more fully expressed in his 1954 book *Motivation and Personality*.[5]

His theory about what motivates humans is depicted in a pyramid diagram with five levels of motivation that describe the layers that human motivation moves through, from lowest to highest. First, our basic physiological needs, then moving up to the most cerebral level of realizing one's true and full potential.

For the names of the five levels, Maslow used the following terms:

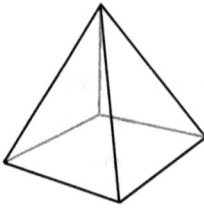

**Level Five**   **Self-Actualization**
**Level Four**   **Esteem**
**Level Three** **Belonging and Love**
**Level Two**   **Safety**
**Level One**   **Physiological Needs**

In its simplistic form, one accomplishes the lower levels before the upper levels. In essence, you need to climb the pyramid.

## PHYSIOLOGICAL NEEDS

The first and bottom level is the largest of all, and as in the Egyptian pyramid, the one with the most weight. Maslow identified the needs of our body: air, water, food, sleep, and sex—all the things that will keep us alive or in the case of sex, keep our species alive. It's what motivates all plants and animals—the need to thrive, survive, and procreate the species.

> ***Think of your body as a temple, not a visitor's center.***
> —ANONYMOUS

## SAFETY NEEDS

The next and second level deals with our environment. It's everything in our physical world, from the surface of our skin going outward. In our ancestral days, the fear of being eaten by a saber-tooth tiger would have been a high-priority environmental fear. Today, saber-tooth tigers are extinct, but our motivation to feel safe in our surroundings is no different. We need shelter from the elements, laws that govern our world, a means to provide a living for ourselves, and the freedom to move about safely.

> **The earth doesn't belong to us. We're merely custodians for a fraction of time.**
> —UNKNOWN

## LOVE AND BELONGING NEEDS

In the third level, we leave the physical world and move into our consciousness. We're social animals: we need to feel a sense of belonging in the world and emotional connections with others. Interpersonal relationships motivate our behavior so that we reach out and connect with others. Friendships, tribes, trusts, acceptance, giving affection, and receiving affection all lead to love. We need to love and be loved.

> **There is nothing on this earth more to be prized than true friendship.**
> —THOMAS AQUINAS, DOMINICAN FRIAR

## ESTEEM NEEDS

The fourth level is also part of our consciousness. Maslow classified this into two categories: esteem for oneself that includes dignity, achievements or skills, and esteem, the desire for respect, prestige, and acknowledgment for one's accomplishments.

> **Self-esteem is the reputation we acquire with ourselves.**
> —NATHANIEL BRANDEN, AMERICAN PSYCHOTHERAPIST

## NEED FOR SELF-ACTUALIZATION

Finally, the fifth level is the desire to become everything you are capable of becoming: your full potential realized. It's the blazing willingness to become the most you can be.

> **Self-actualized people are independent**
> **of the good opinion of others.**
> —WAYNE DYER, AMERICAN SELF-HELP AUTHOR

Although the hierarchy of needs follows an order, Maslow went on to note these needs are somewhat flexible. The hierarchy may ebb and flow in importance. At times, one might have a higher demand for self-esteem over love. We don't fit neatly into these specific levels, as most behavior contains a variety of motivations.

For example, clothing serves to protect our body and therefore falls into protection from our environment in level two, safety. Clothing can also be a means of self-expression, and then dually falls into level four, esteem. Maslow's levels are not precise cuts into our personalities, but rather a guide to question what encompasses our life.

> *It is quite true that man lives by bread alone—when there*
> *is no bread. But what happens to man's desires when there*
> *is plenty of bread and when his belly is chronically filled?*
> *At once, other (and "higher") needs emerge and these,*
> *rather than physiological fits of hunger, dominate the*

*organism. And when these, in turn, are satisfied, again new (and still "higher") needs emerge and so on. This is what we mean by saying that the basic human needs are organized into a hierarchy of relative prepotency.*
—ABRAHAM MASLOW, "A THEORY OF HUMAN MOTIVATION,"
PSYCHOLOGY REVIEW

In the end, a person is always growing and discovering more about themselves. We're not static in our pursuits. Each of us is unique as far as what motivates us. For some, it's the arts, literature, the creative process, or raising a family. Still others are more motivated within the corporate setting or boardroom, by athletics, or by science.

*The body is a vehicle, driven by the mind, fueled by the spirit.*
—SISTER MADONNA BUDER, OLDEST WOMAN TO COMPLETE AN
IRONMAN TRIATHLON, (COMPLETED OVER FORTY IRONMAN RACES)

# NEEDS, WANTS AND DESIRES

Maslow expressed a *need* as something you can't live without, such as air, water, food, sleep and shelter. Needs are absolute and mandatory to sustain our life.

A *want* is something that you don't need. For example, you may think you need a car but you could walk, or take public transportation. Your life doesn't depend on having a car. We want a car to make our commute easier. Most things we want are to improve the quality of our life, and therefore, a want is considered a mild form of desire.

The characteristic of want is that it's forever changing. For example, I want chocolate cookies and tomorrow maybe I'll want potato chips. I want the latest cell phone even though my current cell phone works just fine. Wants fluctuate, but mostly wants are for pleasure, to make our lives better, or for some convenience.

A *desire* is much stronger. Desire can deeply fuel our motivation, actions and decisions. Worthy or unworthy, desire motivates us to attain or possess something, someone or some accomplishment. It could be a worthy desire, like to become a scientist to cure cancer. Or an unworthy desire, like owning the exclusive rights to a life-saving drug, then jacking the price sky-high to get rich.

Professor Steven Reiss of Ohio State University has found that there are sixteen basic desires. The desires are power, independence, curiosity, acceptance, order, saving, honor, idealism, social contact, family, status, vengeance, romance, eating, physical exercise, and tranquility. "These desires are what drive our everyday actions and make us who we are," Reiss said. "What makes individuals unique is the combination and ranking of these desires." [6]

What combination of desires drive you?

> *Desire is the starting point of all achievement,*
> *not a hope, not a wish, but a keen pulsating*
> *desire which transcends everything.*
> —NAPOLEON HILL, AMERICAN AUTHOR

With desire comes action and decisions that can sometimes snowball into big ideas that motivate us to achieve overwhelming accomplishments, wealth, health, and happiness. No matter how great or small, every decision and action affect some piece of this puzzle.

> *There is a choice you have to make in*
> *everything you do. So keep in mind that in the*
> *end, the choice you make, makes you.*
> —JOHN WOODEN, BASKETBALL COACH

## CHANGING THE WORLD BY MAKING YOUR BED

In 2014, Admiral William H. McRaven provided the commencement address for the graduating class at the University of Texas at Austin. He noted the university's motto, "What starts here changes the world."

Building on that motto, Admiral McRaven added, "If you want to change the world, start off by making your bed."

He explained that accomplishing this simple task will give you a small sense of pride, and that small sense of pride will lead you to the next task and the future.

The little things in life matter.

"If you can't do the little things right, you'll never be able to do the big things right."[7]

For every action, there's an outcome or immediate reward. With daily repetition, these actions become habits, and habits have long-term negative or positive consequences.

The immediate reward of making your bed provides a small sense of pride. According to Admiral McRaven, the daily routine of making your bed could give you the discipline you need to go out and change the world.

In order to achieve the big stuff, you have to start with the little stuff. This book is a road map to help you organize and rethink the little stuff. It's the doable little decisions that will guide you to your own remarkable life.

*Climbing to the top demands strength, whether it is to the top of Mount Everest or to the top of your career.*
—A. P. J. ABDUL KALAM, ELEVENTH PRESIDENT OF INDIA

Many years ago, I trekked partway up Mount Everest. The months leading up to my sojourn, I trained brutally hard, doing the elliptical stair-stepper with a loaded backpack. My pencil-thin thighs were burning to build up strength for the trek. I bought the appropriate gear: boots, clothes with breathable fabrics, polar fleece jackets, and waterproof outerwear. I was geared up and prepped up. It was hard going at such high altitudes, but step by step, I climbed.

Climbing Maslow's pyramid takes the same amount of effort—maybe not the same physical toll, but a mental toll. It takes focus, dedication, determination. As you ascend Maslow's pyramid, stop along the way and allow yourself to rethink your desires, actions and decisions. Ask yourself if your actions and desires serve the life you want. For me, trekking Mount Everest and Maslow's pyramid provided watershed moments.

> **A *watershed moment is a turning point*, the exact moment that changes the direction of an activity or situation ... a dividing point, from which things will never be the same. It is considered momentous.[8]**

It was all the little watershed moments that propelled me through decisions, and for me, everything in this book affected me in momentous ways. The small incremental decisions made the momentous doable.

# PART ONE

---

# On the Inside

*I stand in awe of my body.*

—HENRY DAVID THOREAU

*To keep the body in good health is a duty... otherwise we*
*shall not be able to keep our mind strong and clear.*

—BUDDHA

## WHAT MAKES LIFE?

The discovery of what makes life possible started with a failed vaudeville writer. Vaudeville, first popularized in the 1800s, was a music hall that hosted small theatrical acts. It was the failure of Claude Bernard whose dream of vaudeville was dismissed when theater owners thought he had no talent.

He turned to medicine and became a physician. He hated the idea of dealing with people's illnesses and decided to do something most thought revolting. Through dissection he studied the human anatomy in an attempt to find out how the body worked—how life worked. By the 1850s his achievements were identified as extraordinary, bringing him worldwide fame unmatched by any scientist of that time. By his death in 1878, his home country of France accorded him the highest honor possible, a public funeral.

The wonders of our body never cease to unfold. Our discoveries continue today with the breakthrough of genetic engineering, growing organs in a lab, curing cancers with bacteria, and the latest discover, the interstitium, interconnect fluid filled sacs under the skin—now identified as the largest organ of the body.

In the coming section, Part One: On the Inside, we will delve into what's on the inside of our bodies and the science of life itself. From our molecular systems to whole body function, we'll discover the small relevant changes that can power you to improve and advance your body's state of health and wellbeing. Oxygen, hydration, food, sleep, and sex, are the five basic needs but in this section, you will discover they're far from basic. They're complex and the most important factors in keeping you alive.

## CHAPTER THREE

# Your Body's Missing Owner's Manual

*It is health that is real wealth and*
*not pieces of gold and silver.*
—MAHATMA GANDHI

## THE STORY OF MISS SUSAN

It was a charity luncheon. Someone I had never met sat next to me and introduced herself.

Susan is a charmer. She has beautiful, sparkling blue eyes that just invite you to tell her your life's story. They also reveal a woman who's got a few good stories of her own. Susan had just retired. Her son had finished his residency, a doctor no less. He graduated without student loans, as Susan and her husband had worked hard to make that happen.

I was able to retire early as well. And having been there, I said, "I have some valuable advice for you." Susan perked up, leaned in and said, "Tell me."

And just like that, I knew we'd be lifelong friends. I was the fountain of wisdom to the land she had never seen before: retirement land. She had been married, supported her hubby through medical school, raised their son, and then supported her son through medical school as well. Her life was just beginning to be her own, and she was looking to me to guide her on to the road ahead. Years later, she would recount the advice I gave her that sunny, spring day and remind me it was the best advice she had ever received.

My advice was simple.

I told her to join a gym, hire a personal trainer, and for the next six months say no to everything anyone asked her to do. This may seem like odd advice—to say no to whatever demanded her brainpower.

I went on to explain that she had been in her head all her life. Like the hamster on the wheel, critically thinking about her business, dealing with clients, pushing papers, dealing with invoices, phone calls, emails, then more invoices, phone calls, emails—in a rinse-and-repeat head trip. Making hundreds of daily decisions connected with performing her business, meeting family demands, creating grocery lists, and arranging schedules had become her daily habit. This habituated continuous thinking left little time for much else. Her retirement would be the opportunity to get out of her head and hit the reset button. My advice was to take some time for herself—and the best place to begin is with the body.

Because she was a proven critical thinker, people would be asking her to join boards, head up the book club, organize outings or do some other brain-draining chore. I explained if she cluttered her life with more thinking activities, the new retirement glow would quickly fade into the drudgery of just another job—an unpaid job this time. It would be the job of scheduling all those brain-draining activities.

This was her time. "It's a matter of putting your brain on hold to put your body first," I told her, "and take advantage of the time as a gift to do what is best for your body and your soul." This was it: the opportunity to recharge the body and put her physical health as a priority for the rest of her life.

Every day is a new beginning to do what's best for you. Waking up is a new opportunity to get in touch with the most essential part of your being—your own body. It all begins with the body. Maslow put the body first for a reason. When you make time for the body to be its best, it'll help make everything else fall into place.

*The mind's first step to self-awareness*
*must be through the body.*

—GEORGE SHEEHAN, PHYSICIAN AND ATHLETE

## THE BODY, IT BEGINS HERE

You have to get out of your head to make room for your body.

The physical body is so complicated. There are interconnected bio systems that do amazing things to keep us alive. An adult has about 100 trillion cells organized into fifteen major organs (brain, heart, lungs, spleen, liver, stomach, kidneys, gallbladder, pancreas, bladder, appendix, large and small intestines, male and female genitals, and our skin) all supported by two hundred and six distinct bones, and encased in an architecturally beautiful support system of over six hundred skeletal muscles, all contained neatly within our largest of organs, our layer of protective skin. Our body's design is absolute perfection—a gift from the universe as well as our parents.

*There is but one temple in the universe,*
*and that is the body of man.*

—NOVALIS, GERMAN PHILOSOPHER

Acknowledging this gift of being here is the start of a journey through all the body's needs. As Maslow pointed out, the physical body has five basic instincts, urges, or requirements for purposing its survival and propagation:

Air, water, food, sleep, and sex.

The first four are needed to maintain your individual life, and the fifth to sustain the species as a whole. In the next few chapters, we'll look deeper into these five basic needs. You'll discover new, life-changing techniques to transform your daily habits and power your very existence.

## CHAPTER FOUR

# Breath In, Breath Out... Repeat as Needed

*A human being is only breath and shadow.*

—SOPHOCLES, ANCIENT GREEK PLAYWRIGHT

Breathing is our first and most basic need.

When we enter the world from our mother's body, everyone in the birthing room holds their collective breath—waiting for the newly born babe to take its first inhalation, inflating its tiny lungs, followed by a good, wailing cry. It's that first breath that ignites the very flame of life within us, independent of our mother's womb, breathing on our own.

Unless you've studied breathing, you probably take the whole breathe in, breathe out thing for granted. You may think, What's the big deal?

There's more to breathing than you would think and there's an art to forming good breathing habits that will change your life.

In my first career, I was a respiratory therapist in the open-heart cardiac post-op surgical unit. It was my job to monitor the ventilators that did the breathing for the post-op open-heart patients until they were stable and could breathe on their own. I worked in other units—head trauma, neo-natal, the burn unit—and I was part of the "code blue" emergency response team. It was my job to begin resuscitation when a patient was in cardiopulmonary arrest.

I loved my work in the hospital. I felt I was helping people and their families at one of the most critical times of their lives. I felt my profession in the hospital put me at ground zero for keeping people alive.

Ever since then, I've been an observer of the breath. How you breathe can affect your overall health, ability to think, and energy level. Your ability to breathe can be affected by something as small as your posture or as big as the quality of the air around you.

Meandering through the day, the average person breathes about sixteen times a minute, nine hundred sixty times per hour, twenty-three thousand times a day, and over eight million times a year. When you do the math, it's a staggering amount, and you can see the importance just by the fact you're doing it all the time.

Depending on our body's oxygen needs, breathing is automatically regulated. For example, during exercising, levels of carbon dioxide levels in the blood increase, activating the carotid and aortic bodies. Those bodies send nerve impulses to the respiratory center of the brain to kick it up and tell you to breathe more often and deeper. "Ay Captain Kirk, we're giving her all she's got!"

On the other hand, if you only want to make a dent on the couch, zone out, and nap through reruns of *Star Trek*, your breath slows and becomes shallow. Your aerobic needs have decreased to a level that would keep a potato alive—a couch potato.

> *The only reason I would take up jogging is so*
> *that I could hear heavy breathing again.*
> —ERMA BOMBECK, HUMORIST

Our autonomic nervous system is like the body's backup generator. If you get knocked unconscious, the body's functions don't temporarily fail. We don't have to worry that our cardiovascular, digestive, and respiratory function will temporarily shut off.

The autonomic nervous system regulates certain functions, like breathing, digestion, heart pumping, and blood flow. It's like an autopilot setting—it just happens. The breath is part of the system, but to a certain extent the breath can be controlled, making it unique.

You can hold your breath until you turn blue as a Smurf, but at some point (after one to three minutes, if you're the average person), you'll be driven to take that revitalizing gasp. The gasp is the auto part, but holding your breath for a while is the control part.

You have no control over your cardiovascular or digestive systems. You cannot stop your heart for a while or stop your kidneys from turning that last cup of coffee into urine. But the breath is different. Learning to control your breathing patterns can be beneficial in addressing stress, calming the mind, changing your emotions, and igniting the flow of critical thinking.

## BREATH IS THE KING OF THE MIND

Illusionist and endurance artist David Blaine once appeared on *The Oprah Winfrey Show* to attempt to break the record for holding his breath. Submerged in an acrylic chamber filled with water, he did the seemingly impossible and held his breath for over seventeen minutes. This feat put him in *The Guinness Book of World Records*. To prepare for his performance, he inhaled pure oxygen for twenty-three minutes to over-oxygenate his entire body, and then calmed his mind to a deep meditative state.

This is akin to the yogic practice of pranayama, pronounced "pra-na-ya-ma." In yogic Sanskrit, pranayama means lengthening of the prana, or breath. The word is broken down as *prana*, meaning life force or vital energy, in particular the breath, and *ayama*, to lengthen or extend. Through breath control, it's possible to still the mind and attain higher states of awareness. Widely considered the father of modern yoga, Mr. BKS Iyengar demonstrates in a YouTube video an inhalation that takes fifty-five seconds to complete. The exhalation takes approximately thirty-three seconds. He states, "The breath is the king of the mind."

Deepening your breath tricks your brain cells into thinking you are in a calm state. Yoga students have practiced this for years, but recent research identified 175 brain cells that do not regulate the breath, but spy on breath patterns instead, then loop this information back to the brainstem. The researchers found that changing the pattern of your breath makes it possible to reverse-engineer your mood. For example, slowing the breath calms the brain. "*If something's impairing or accelerating your breathing, you need to know right away,*" said Dr. Mark Krasnow, biochemistry professor at the Stanford University School of Medicine. "*These 175 neurons, which tell the rest of the brain what's going on, are absolutely critical.*"[9]

These neurons pick up your various breathing patterns, from the shallow breathing during sleep to the forceful deep breathing during aerobic exercise. They link your breath to relaxation. The oxygen levels of the brain are tied to the level of the neurotransmitter serotonin. Serotonin is the hormone that helps us be alert and can elevate our mood. Through breathing exercises and elongating the breath, you can increase the hormonal and hemispherical balance of the brain. This can result in greater relaxation, and allows the brain's intuitive spirit and nonlinear thinking to flow more smoothly.

Whoa. Who thought your breath is the Dr. Feelgood of your body? And it's all free with positive side-effects.

Traditional Chinese medicine believes whichever nostril you habitually breathe through most tells you which side of the brain you favor. For example, if you breathe more through your right nostril than your left, you might favor more left-brain thinking. Right-brain thinking is believed to be more artistic and creative. Left-brain thinking is believed to be more analytical and methodical. To rebalance the hemispheres of the brain and facilitate cross-hemispherical thinking, or the whole-brain thinking, Chinese medicine recommends this technique:

1. Hold one nostril closed with your thumb.
2. Slowly breathe in and out through the opposite nostril for five seconds.
3. Repeat on the other side.

Balancing the brain improves mental clarity. You'll slow down your brain waves from beta to alpha, thus facilitating intuitive, inspired thought.

That explains my sudden burst in left-brain thinking after the surgery to fix my deviated septum.

## BREATH AND MEDITATION

The gym I go to is on the lower floors of a very stylish office building. There's a thirty-foot-long landscaped area between the street parking and entrance that has a small grove of eucalyptus trees and cedar bushes. With the smells of earth and cedar, it's a little slice of heaven. As if I've entered a shrine, my brain immediately calms. I always stop there and just breathe.

You can also perform a breathing meditation anywhere. Just stop wherever you are and focus on the pace and depth of your inhalations and exhalations. This will become your go-to salvation for slowing down the speed of life and relaxing.

Meditation can also improve the brain, even if you give it only one minute. During meditation, the frontal cortex tends to go offline. This area of the brain is involved with reasoning, planning, emotions, and self-awareness. It also processes sensory information about the surrounding world. Meditation—going off-line—gives you a respite. This may very well be the reason many monasteries and meditation centers are located in natural surroundings. Nothing supports opening the mind and heart like the beauty, tranquility, and silence of the natural world. For me, the landscaped median between the street parking and entrance of my gym serves as an oasis in a desert of concrete.

> **Breathing is central to every aspect of meditation training. It's a wonderful place to focus on training the mind to be calm and concentrated.**
> —JON KABAT-ZINN, CREATOR OF THE STRESS REDUCTION CLINIC

## BREATH AND THE HEART

*September 11, 2001, Los Angeles, California*

It was too early for the phone to be ringing. It was Jack's son. He told us to turn on the TV.

We sat in horror, watching the second plane hit the second tower of the World Trade Center. Moments later, one by one, both towers imploded, collapsing to the ground. I was shaken to my core. I felt someone had ripped out my throat, pounded my heart into hamburger, and drained my body of all blood. The following nights, I was haunted by the horror of those people who jumped to their deaths rather than choosing to be burnt alive.

The Saturday after the tragedy, I was scheduled for a daylong advanced yoga workshop with an advanced Iyengar yoga instructor on the West

Coast, Manuso Manos. He was only in town every couple of months, and I got one of the coveted spots. I checked my email for the class cancellation. Undoubtedly, I thought, the world will stop, as all America was heartbroken. It was as if the entire United States was covered with a blanket of black grief. But by Saturday morning, there was still no email or phone call cancelling the seminar. I put on my yoga togs and just went. I figured it had to be cancelled, but I would get a couple of much-needed hugs from my fellow yoga friends.

Manuso was there, and the class was on. Huh? How could I do this advanced yoga class with my body in such a state of grief? The fibers of my muscles were locked up, my stomach in knots, I couldn't breathe, and my head just hung in sorrow. I felt as if someone had stabbed me right in my heart. But Manuso was there. Amazingly, everyone who had signed up *just showed up*. We were all in the collective consciousness of needing each other.

Manuso had everyone lie down, back flat on the floor, knees bent, and just breathe. At first, I felt crippled just trying to lie there. He went on to explain how, now more than ever, we needed yoga. That yoga would help us ease the pain of grief in our body, open our hearts and be able to send love into the world again. After a while, I felt the ball of sadness start to ease, my soul opened and I felt I could breathe again.

The class went on, but the sweat-dripping, advanced poses were replaced with restorative poses to open the chest and breathing, lots of breathing. It saved me, pulling me out of a state of deep depression. I left the class feeling I had something to give to the world. I had love in my heart again.

> **When your chest is open, And you're**
> **breathing deeply, it lifts your spirits.**
> —MANDY INGBER, YOGA INSTRUCTOR AND ACTRESS

## AIR SO THICK YOU COULD CHEW IT

📌

Just breathe.
Deeply. Fully.
Consciously.
Breathe.

The oxygenation of our cells powers our body's functions and physical activity. Oxygen deprivation can impair our immune system, causing disease and accelerating the aging process. Our brain uses the highest percentage of the oxygen that we breathe. While our brain makes up 2 percent of our body mass, it uses a whopping 20 percent of the oxygen we inhale.

On Sunday, January 20, 2013, the air quality index in New York City was at 13 on a scale that runs from 0 to 500. The worst pollution in the United States on that day was in Tacoma, Washington, which registered at 91. In the United States, the air quality index considers anything over 200 to be "very unhealthy." At that level, it's recommended people with heart or lung disease, the elderly, and children avoid all outdoor physical activities, and that everyone should avoid prolonged or heavy outdoor exertion.

That same day in Beijing, China, the air quality was an unthinkable 755. Beijing had been experiencing record-low temperatures that led to an increase in burning coal for heat. There's a horseshoe ring of mountains around the city that trapped the pollution from burning coal, pollution from China's booming factories, and car exhaust from China's explosive growth in car ownership. As reported by China's Ministry of Commerce, China Daily, and the World Bank, during this time China was the number one source of carbon emissions worldwide, with China having twenty of the top thirty most polluted cities in the world.

A sequence of factors affects our ability to breathe effectively. It starts with the quality of the air. Then, we must have the physical ability to inhale and expand the chest. The membrane of the lungs must be permeable for the oxygen to transfer into our bloodstream. And finally, the blood delivers oxygen's "life force" to each cell of the entire body.

Take smoking, for example. The smoke irritates and causes swelling of the lung tissues. Over time, these irritants from smoke cause the small sections of the lungs called alveoli to break down into bigger air pockets, thus decreasing the surface area of the lungs. Less surface area means less oxygen can get across the lung's membranes into the bloodstream. This degradation of the lungs' surface impairs your ability to breathe, leading to chronic obstructive pulmonary disease (COPD) or emphysema. Long-term smoking is linked to other chronic diseases, heart disease, and increased risk of cancers. Even as few as two cigarettes a day can cause damage and impair your ability to breath effectively.

Cigarettes also contain micronized amounts of tar and of course, nicotine. The tar deposits are sticky and get lodged in the small alveoli, coating the air pockets and decreasing the lungs' ability to perfuse oxygen even more. The same goes for vaping nicotine or even cannabis oils. The cannabis is in the form of an oil that is then micronized into a vapor you inhale. These oils get stuck in the alveoli as well. You wouldn't breathe the aerosol from a can of vegetable oil used to coat a pan for cooking, so why would it be safe to breathe in oils from cannabis? It's not, and several young adults have landed in intensive care units for critical long-term treatment because of it.

There's a second part to this. The lungs breathe in oxygen to nourish the cells, but in the exhale, they also take the toxic waste of carbon dioxide away. Coating the lungs' membranes with tar, cannabis oil, and the irritants of nicotine not only impair the ability to get nourishing oxygen to the cells but also reduces the body's ability to rid the cells of carbon dioxide. The cells of the body need food, oxygen, and water to survive. In reverse, the cells need to rid the body of waste through urine, feces, and exhaling carbon dioxide. The body is never stagnant in these functions—you can't put them on hold.

Poor air quality creates most lung issues, whether it's from smoking, vaping, or living in an environment where the air is heavily polluted. In 2018, Greenpeace and AirVisual named Gurugram, a suburb of New Delhi in India, as the city with the world's worst air pollution. That year, seven of the top ten cities worldwide with the worst air pollution were in India.[10]

Back in the 1980s, restaurants had smoking sections. Smoke goes where it wants, and a "smoking section" became irrelevant. It was determined secondhand smoke is as toxic as smoking yourself. Public opinion won out, and restaurants, office buildings, and public places eventually became smoke-free environments.

*All things share the same breath—the beast, the tree, the man ... the air shares its spirit with all the life it supports.*
—CHIEF SEATTLE, 1800'S SUQUAMISH AND DUWAMISH CHIEF

No matter where you are, air pollutants are hard to escape. The microscopic particles can be airborne, and because they're lighter than air, they can travel far past the immediate area to affect everyone in the world. These microscopic pollutants can penetrate deep into the respiratory system, damaging the lungs and in turn, the rest of the body.

In March 2011, three Fukushima nuclear reactor blew, the result of a chain-reaction that started with a magnitude 9.0 earthquake. Releasing radioactive particulates into the atmosphere, it was the worst nuclear disaster since Chernobyl in 1986. Dangerous airborne contaminants from the reactors quickly spread, pushing the evacuation zone around the reactors further to an area of 154,000 residents.

Radioactive material continued to seep into the atmosphere and the Pacific Ocean, creating devastating environmental damage to both. As with the smoking section in a restaurant, the spread of the radioactive pollutants continued eastward, hitting the United States three days after the Fukushima disaster. Although the radiation levels detected in US air, water, grass, and milk were purported to be below any level of public and environmental concern, it still happened. The United States is over six-thousand miles away from Japan, over twice the distance from New York to Los Angeles. The distance may have allowed the particulates to dissipate into the atmosphere, spreading the toxicity. That may have been what was reported but it was nonetheless scary for all in the wake of the wave of nuclear fallout.

Whether through second-hand smoke, a nuclear explosion in Japan, or the air pollution over Gurugram, India, we are all connected and breathe the same air. To check the quality of air where you live, most cities have air quality index websites. Another option would be to invest in a whole-home or portable air filtration system.

## WHY SITTING IS THE NEW SMOKING

The actions of breathing can be broken down into a few anatomical movements. When you inhale the diaphragm drops down, the abdomen expands, the ribs move up and apart, and the little intercostal muscles between the ribs stretch. The chest cavity expands, especially the front of the chest, and the lungs fill with air. Posture must be correct to effectuate a full, deep breath. But the problem is 60 to 70 percent of the US population sits at a desk to do their work.

*New Survey: To sit or stand? Almost 70 percent of full time American workers hate sitting, but they do it all day every day.*
—PR NEWSWIRE

"Sitting is more dangerous than smoking, kills more people than HIV, and is more treacherous than parachuting. We are sitting ourselves to death," declares James Levine, a professor of medicine at the Mayo Clinic. "*The chair is out to kill us.*"[11]

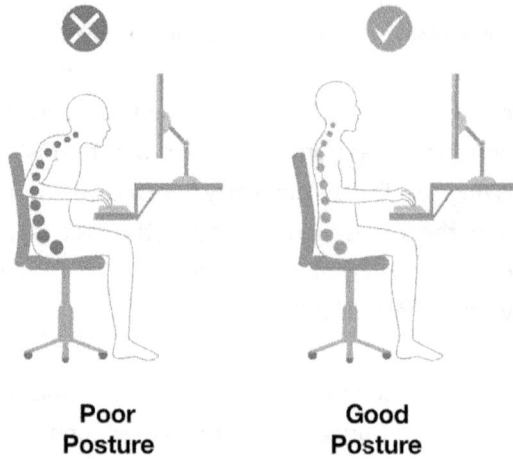

**Poor Posture**    **Good Posture**

**POOR POSTURE CLOSES THE FRONT CHEST DISRUPTING THE LUNGS ABILITY TO INFLATE FULLY.**

Sitting leads to hunching forward and the front body closing down. The front ribs can't move up and apart, and the internal organs are pushing the diaphragm up into the chest. The chest cavity is in a perpetual locked-down, exhaled position, making the chest cavity smaller. As a result, our lungs are squashed, and it's impossible to take a full, deep breath. As with smoking, the ability of the body to get air into the lungs is impaired. Weak breathing means your body, and especially your brain, is not getting the oxygen it needs.

The knowledge I have gained as a respiratory therapist and after years of observing the breath, practicing Iyengar yoga, and countless hours of fitness training have led me to develop a class. The class focuses on postural correction and breathing. I don't like to use the word *fitness or workout* for it, because it's not. The class is meant to unmold my students from the hunched-over, rounded shoulders, closed hips, and neck-jutting-forward effects of sitting and poor posture. When your mother told you, "Pull your shoulders back," she was not giving you the whole picture. It's more profound and more complicated than one move. Posture is head to toes and everything in between.

My students come in shrunken messes and leave taller with their chest open, head erect and fired up with breath. Their brain is alive with a new sense of clarity and they feel great. All because I spend the time on the littlest things, like the intercostal muscles between each rib. Stretching those little muscles gives room for the ribs to move apart and opens the chest. What a difference it would make in everyone's life if we could all take the time to do the same!

# POSTURAL-BASED LUMBAR PAIN

I mention back pain here to bring light to the other complications of sitting and poor posture. Nearly 80 percent of adults experience lower back pain sometime in their life. It's the most common job-related disability and the leading cause of missed days at work.[12] Any pain we experience affects our ability to breath correctly and fully, but with sitting there's more to be concerned about than just our breathing.

Our bodies simply weren't designed to sit all day. It's the lumbar vertebrae and their squishy discs that bear the brunt of sitting. These discs are meant to cushion the vertebrae and support the spine, but the weight of the upper body from sitting creates constant compression and over the years can cause premature discs degeneration and chronic pain. With poor posture your lower back is swayed one way or another creating uneven pressure on the spine that can lead to sciatica, spinal stenosis, and damage to the ligaments and nerves.

Imagine placing a large gumdrop on the table and then stacking sixty pounds of books on top of it. After eight hours, take a look at how the gum drop has held its shape. It's squished. That gum drop did about as well as the discs in your lumbar vertebrae.

It's best not to sit a lot. When you do, take breaks, move the lower back and relieve the pressure on the discs, stretch, and get plenty of exercise.

Above all have good posture that evenly distributes the weight over the entire discs, vertebrae and spine.

If you do sit a lot, then you need habits that support a healthy spine. When it comes to learning physical actions such as good posture techniques, there's a process as to how your brain and body connect. You learn in a sequence of three cues: first, by observing the technique, then listening carefully to the instructions, then by doing it yourself. Then, you repeat the process about a thousand times until your body knows the action. Good posture then becomes your new mindless habit and state of being.

Healthy posture means improved lung capacity, and that means more oxygen to the body and brain. It also decreases postural-based pain; like head and neck strain from looking down at your computer or back pain from sitting improperly. The body becomes more relaxed when the body stacked and aligned, allowing better mental, emotional and physical performance.

Correct your posture with these doable moves:

1. Stand with your arms at your side, face your palms outward and point your thumbs backward. This first move opens the chest by moving your shoulder blades together and down your back.

2. Now, tuck your chin. Look straight ahead, keeping your eyes level to keep your head erect and stacked over the spine.

3. Next, turn your attention to your waistline. Imagine the circumference of your waistline is the rim of a bowl filled with water. Now, roll your tail bone down as if you were going to pour water out the back of the bowl or in other words, out the back of your pants.

4. Engage the abs by sucking the navel backwards to the spine.

5. If performed correctly, you will be standing taller with your chest open and your hips stacked over your feet. Simple. Now enjoy.

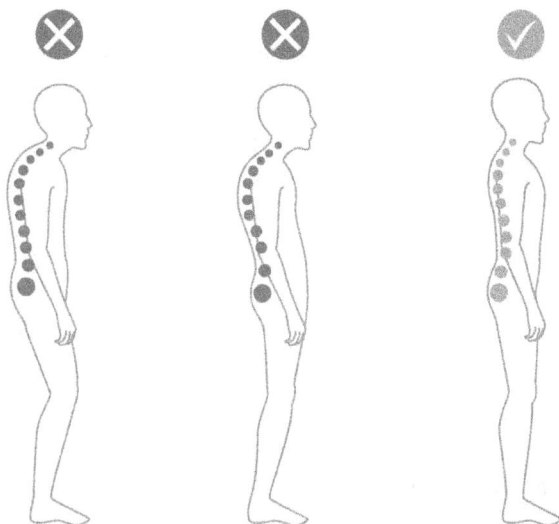

**POOR POSTURE**

**GOOD POSTURE**

## NITRIC OXIDE AND NASAL BREATHING

You have two options. Breathe through your mouth or breathe through your nose. Breathing through the nose filters and adds humidity to the air you take in. Most important, the sinus cavity excretes a gas, nitric oxide. Mixing this gas with the breath aids the transfer of oxygen and carbon dioxide in and out of the cells. Nitric oxide may also provide a defense against specific microorganisms like bacteria and viruses. Although more research would be needed, nitric oxide is believed to play a vital role in biological functions, such as blood flow, immunity, and neurotransmitters, including the formation of memory.

Vibrations from humming or making a buzzing sound increases the release of nitric oxide by as much as fifteen times. Breathing through the nose adds nitric oxide from the sinuses and oxygenates the blood about 10 to 15 percent more than breathing though the mouth.[13]

Most yoga practices begin with chanting the sacred syllable, *om*, three times. *Om* is pronounced "aum," and the three times honors your past, present, and future. *Om* is believed to be the basic sound of the universe, and chanting it will physically tune us into that sound. Chanting *om* vibrates at a frequency of 432 Hz, believed to be the same vibrational frequency in all things throughout nature. The ancient yogis somehow knew all this, and science has caught up to them and proven it.

Next time you're stuck in mind-numbing traffic, remember the yogis. Take a deep breath and let it rip: "Aaaauuuummmm."

## BOX BREATHING

Laird Hamilton and his wife, Gabby Reece, developed a lifestyle training program, XPT, where they teach breathwork as part of their program. As a master of big wave surfing, Laird knows the ability to hold your breath underwater will save your life. He also knows practicing breath control forces the body to utilize the oxygen more efficiently.

One of their technique is called "box breathing," where the length of each inhale is matched with a hold, and each exhale paired with a hold. Simply put, it's a 1:1:1:1 ratio: inhale for four seconds, hold for four seconds, exhale for four seconds, hold for four seconds. After a while, you can increase the time periods. 8-8-8-8, 12-12-12-12, and so on. The practice pushes you to discover your limits. Breath control, like this practice teaches, helps you move past the fight-or-flight tendency into a relaxed response and the ability to breathe through it.[14]

The root words of *inspiration* are *in* and *spire*, which together means "to breathe in." To be inspired is to be full of the breath of life. Whenever you notice your breathing is compromised, stop, and deliberately take a long, slow, deep breath.

**I'm thankful to be breathing, on this side of the grass. Whatever comes, comes.**

—RON PERLMAN, ACTOR

---

## CHAPTER SUMMARY

☑ **Meditation**

Even five minutes will make a difference, and it's doable. Can't quite get the hang of it? The box breathing method is an excellent place to start. Breathing meditation can relieve anxiety, stress, and tension in the body leading to greater inner peace, focus, and mind control.

☑ **Air Quality**

Be conscious of your environmental air. If you live in an area with significant air pollution, consider moving, having a few air purifiers, or at times, wearing a mask. It's your lungs and your life. I always have a paper mask that conveniently fits in my purse. It comes in handy, especially on flights with people coughing. Starting a vacation off catching someone's flu virus is no fun.

☑ **Nitric Oxide Nasal Breathing**

The breath starts with the nasal passages where nitric oxide is added to the air. If you wake up in the morning with dry mouth and congestion, you may be bypassing the nasal sinuses and breathing through your mouth all night, or worse, snoring. Nothing can irritate a spouse or bed partner more than being awakened by snoring.

A way not to wake the snoring beast inside you is a little trick I learned—tape your mouth shut. Not the entire mouth—this isn't a gag order—just a small half-inch piece of paper tape down the center, from the top lip to the bottom lip, as a gentle reminder to breathe through your nose. Okay, it's not your sexiest look but you'll wake more refreshed, and so will your bed companion.

The same goes for the daytime—practice using your nasal passages. When I have a training session at home, I often use the same tape technique. Breathing through the nose is a vital part of the breath process. If the whole tape-your-mouth thing is a little scary, hold a piece of paper between your lips as you train. This will also force you to breathe through your nose instead of your mouth.

## ☑ Postural Corrections

Good posture will open the chest and improve your ability to breathe effectively. It'll help prevent spine issues down the line. It can also make you appear and feel more confident.

CHAPTER FIVE

# Lifeblood for You and the Planet

*Water is life's matter and matrix, mother, and medium.*
*There is no life without water.*
—ALBERT SZENT-GYORGYI, HUNGARIAN BIOCHEMIST,
1937 NOBEL PRIZE IN PHYSIOLOGY

Clean water is vital to the survival of life. You can live about three days without water before the body starts to shut down. Most major cities in the United States have successfully piped water to each household, so we usually don't have to venture any further than the kitchen sink to drink clean, fresh water. We don't have to dig wells, tote water in buckets, or think much about it. It's just magically there. We take having fresh water for granted.

Water: every person and every living thing needs it, which makes water management, infrastructure, and waste disposal critical to the safety and development of all habitats, communities, the nation and the planet.

For example, the state of California has one of the most complicated water management systems, and has been called the most hydrolog-ically altered landmass on the planet. All to get life-saving water to its residents, farm animals, wildlife, wetlands, rivers, and support the vast agriculture industries. To get a drink of water in Los Angeles, your water most likely traveled over 400 miles.

> *I grew up during the war years in a tiny cottage with no electricity. Water for washing was pumped from a pond, my brother and I had to fetch drinking water from a tap at the end of the lane, and light was from candles, paraffin lamps, and our nightly log fire.*
> —HELEN CRAIG, CHILDREN'S BOOK AUTHOR AND ILLUSTRATOR

The song popularized in the 1970s, *It Never Rains in Southern California*, holds true today as the average rain fall is less then fifteen inches per year, a miniscule amount compared to the water demands of California's forty million people. That's why in order for Southern California to survive, 70 percent of its water comes from the northern third of the state as precipitation from snow. Over 80 percent of all California's water demands are in the southern two-thirds of the state. Water management engineers had to be creative about how to move massive amounts of water from the north to the south and developed the aqueduct systems, a vast, complicated network of tunnels and pipes that convey water throughout California.

Why is this important? Life doesn't exist without water, even if you need to move mountains to get it. California is dependent on pipes, like arteries and veins throughout the human body to supply blood, the aqueduct system supplies life to all California. But California's system of water also affects everyone in the United States and the world.

California produces two-thirds of the nation's fruits and vegetables, and the state makes more money from agriculture than any other state in the country. California almonds account for 80 percent of all global almond production. Each nut takes a gallon of water to produce, accounting for 10 percent of the state's agricultural water use—more than the water used by the entire population of Los Angeles and San Francisco combined.

Surprisingly, almonds are not the most water-intensive crop. That would be alfalfa. 70 percent of the alfalfa is grown for feed for the cattle and dairy industries. In fact, according the *Wall Street Journal* article, "A fast-food quarter-pounder costs $3, and 1,300 gallons of water. That's how much it takes, per burger, to hydrate the cow, grow its food, and process its carcass. By contrast, a loaf of bread uses up 150 gallons, and milk requires just 65."[15]

I use California's aqueducts as an example to show how complicated water truly is. We turn a tap, water comes out and our user experience stops there. You need to look further and see the impact of water on all your choices.

I'll use California again for another example regarding our responsibility towards habitat preservation and our environment. Water use in California is roughly 50 percent environmental for maintaining rivers and wetlands, 40 percent agricultural, for both animal and plant, and 10 percent urban, for human use.

Over the century, 90 percent of all California's wetlands have been destroyed, filled in, or plowed under, so preserving what's left is vital to maintain any semblance of wildlife population. The Central Valley, once millions of acres of wetlands that hosted the migration patterns of birds and other endemic species, now grows most of the nation's fruits and vegetables. California has more native species than any other state, and a large number of them aren't found anywhere else in the world. For us to survive, these plants and animals need to survive as part of our humanity and culture. By preserving habitats and wetlands, wildlife comes back, and species thrive.

*The greatness of a nation and its moral progress can be judged by the way its animals are treated.*
—MAHATMA GANDHI

Earth is the only planet in the solar system that hosts life as we know it, all because of water. While 70 percent of the earth is covered in water, most is ocean saline-based water, and less than 2.5 percent is drinkable freshwater. Even then, less than 1 percent of freshwater is accessible, with the rest trapped in glaciers and snowfields. Water is a precious commodity we tend to take for granted, especially since it just shows up when we turn the faucet tap on.

Everything on the planet is dependent on water.

# PUREST WATER

My hometown of Independence, Missouri, is a suburb of Kansas City, Missouri. It's known as the home of President Harry Truman, and the gateway to the West for the pioneers who crossed the Overland Trail. Joseph Smith, founder of the Mormon church, once proclaimed it was where the Garden of Eden was located in biblical times. All true trivia, but more surprising, it's also known to have some of the best-tasting water in the world.

For the last seven year, Berkley Springs International Water Tasting competition, the largest water competition in the world, has proclaimed the water of Independence to be the third-best tasting water in the world. That's because Independence's water source is mostly from groundwater, which is of a higher quality than surface water from rivers or reservoirs. Groundwater is from water that, as it trickles down through the earth, collects minerals, and treating groundwater for consumption is a more consistent process.

Arthur Von Wiesenberger, a "watermaster," headed up the taste tests and pointed out that the importance of how water tastes is often overlooked. "I've been told that drinking tap water in New Orleans is like jumping into a swimming pool with your mouth open," said Von Wiesenberger. "It's such a fascinating subject because we take it for granted. Benjamin Franklin said we only know the worth of water when the well is dry."[16]

Most tap water in the United States is deemed safe to drink, but there are exceptions. In 2014, the residents of Flint, Michigan, discovered brown sludge when they turned on their faucets. The city is currently working to replace its old lead pipes. Many cities face aging infrastructure and lead leaching into the drinking water supply. You can check with your local water bureau to learn more about your tap water's quality. You can also purchase a water filtration system that can fit under the kitchen or bathroom counter. Most hook in-line with existing water outlets and require no new plumbing. The filtration systems vary in contaminates they can filter out, so you will have to research their performance. These under-counter filtration systems range in price, but most are around one hundred to two hundred dollars. They will filter out the significant contaminants and provide you with better-quality drinking water at your kitchen or bathroom sink.

*I try to start drinking water as soon as*
*my feet hit the floor in the morning.*
—MARY KAY ANDREWS, BESTSELLING AUTHOR

## WATER POISONING

Depending on the part, the human body ranges in water content from 55 to 85 percent—even something as hard as our bones have a water content of about 30 percent. All cells, organs, and body fluids need water to function, but there's a limit.

Water intoxication is when you drink more water than your kidneys can filter, diluting the electrolytes in your blood. When the sodium level is diluted and falls into the danger zone, it's called hyponatremia.

Through osmosis, sodium acts as a pumping regulator for balancing of fluids inside and outside of the cells. When sodium levels drop outside the cell, fluids shift and move into the cell, causing the cells to swell. It's these electrolytes that maintain an osmotic gradient between various cells that can regulate your body's hydration and blood pH that are critical for nerve and muscle function.

In 2002, some participants of the Boston Marathon provided blood samples prerace and postrace to determine risk factors for hyponatremia. Of those who offered usable samples, 13 percent of the runners had hyponatremia at the end of the race. The dangers of overhydrating became apparent when a twenty-eight-year-old runner collapsed during the race and died two days later. Since then, marathon organizers have tightened runners' qualifications and given guidelines for hydration during the race. More marathon runners have died from over-hydration than from dehydration. In fact, no one has died from dehydration in a marathon.[17]

Symptoms of overhydration can be similar to dehydration, mistakenly leading people to drink more and more water. Symptoms include nausea, vomiting, headache, and a general feeling of malaise.

According to the American Chemistry Society, it would take about six liters of water to kill a 165-pound person. And unfortunately, this sort of death by drinking can be a tragic end to those who challenge themselves to water-drinking contests and among athletes who overhydrate while training. Some seasoned athletes have gone so far as to weigh themselves before and after exercise, concluding any weight loss was from fluid lost through sweat.

Paracelsus, a sixteenth-century scientist, came up with the concept that everything can be a poisonous substance for humans—it just depends on the dosing. Even something as vital as water to the human body, if overdone, can be deadly. We'll talk about adequate daily water needs in a moment, but first let's talk about timing.

## BEST TIME TO DRINK WATER

Mornings can be rough. You've probably woken up to dry mouth, foggy brain, and drowsiness. Throughout the night, you've been sweating and expelling vapor through your breath, and most likely you've had to get up to go to the bathroom to urinate. All this has depleted the fluid content in your body. Since water seeks its own gravitational level, when you get out of bed in the morning and stand up, your brain is drained of fluid, possibly making you lightheaded, irritable, sleepy, or even giving you a slight headache. No wonder we wake up cranky—your brain is running on empty.

*A reduction of 4 to 5 percent in body water will result in a decline of 20 to 30 percent in work performance.*
—HELEN ANDREWS GUTHRIE, INTRODUCTORY NUTRITION

The brain is about 80 percent water and floats inside the skull, but with the loss of fluids throughout the night, your brain may be dry-docked. Symptoms include low blood pressure as your body's fluid content is low, dry mouth, dry skin, fatigue, muscle cramping, constipation, chills, and more.

The optimal time to power-drink some water is first thing in the morning before breakfast, and before that first cup of coffee. When your stomach is empty, drink a couple of glasses of water. This will help cleanse the colon, increasing the efficiency of the intestine to absorb nutrients, and it may help flush out any toxins. Constipation is related to dehydration in the colon. When your body is adequately hydrated, things flow more smoothly.

Replenishing the fluid content of the body has so many benefits. Your organs are rehydrated and can function more efficiently. It can jump-start your brain by increasing blood flow and oxygen, making you more alert and awake. When your brain doesn't have enough water, it can't function properly, leading to headaches, inflammation, fatigue, and possibly even anxiety. When you're hit by the mid-day slump, instead of reaching for another cup of coffee, try rehydrating your brain with water.

*Drinking water is like washing out your insides. The water will cleanse the system, fill you up, decrease your caloric load, and improve the function of all your tissues.*

—KEVIN R. STONE, STONE RESEARCH FOUNDATION

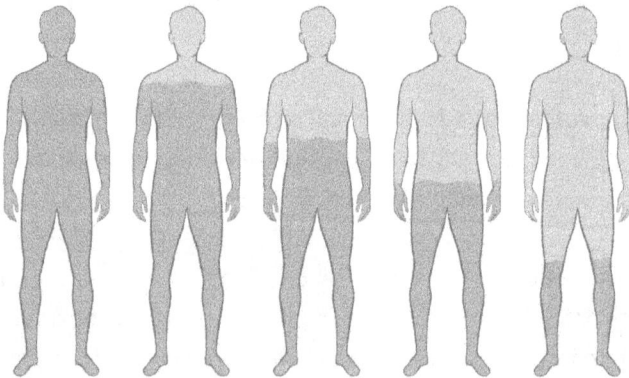

Water is lost throughout the night through evaporation, respiration, perspiration and urination. When you wake and stand up, the loss of water affects your brain the most.

## WATER VS. BEVERAGES

The body relies on water for survival—plain old H2O and *not* beverages loaded with sugar, caffeine, or alcohol.

The exact amount of water the body needs is highly individual. It depends on the physical condition of the person, the amount of physical activity, and the environmental temperature, altitude, and humidity.

For example, people in hotter climates who sweat more will require higher water intake than those in colder climates. If you're running a marathon versus watching the marathon on TV, your hydration needs will be vastly different.

There are believers in the eight glasses of water a day maxim, which can be a basic starting guideline. An individual's level of thirst can also provide a simple guide for how much water they require. If you want to calculate fluid consumption based on your weight, the general rule is to drink between half an ounce to an ounce of water for each pound you weigh. A woman who weighs about one hundred thirty pounds would drink between sixty-five to one hundred thirty ounces of water or fluids a day or between eight to sixteen cups. Because water and beverages come in twelve-ounce sizes, you'll have to make the mathematical adjustment. Most standard glass drinkware or reusable water bottles come in twelve-ounce sizes or larger.

We also get fluids not only from drinking water and other beverages but from the foods we eat. Most food naturally contains water. Fruits, vegetables, and even meats have water content, and we meet approximately 20 percent of our fluid needs with the foods we eat.[18]

Beverages are the fluids we drink other than water. There are natural beverages, like milk and fruit juices. And there are manufactured beverages, like ones enhanced with vitamins, carbonation, antioxidants, performance enhancers, herbal supplements, and yes, I have even seen waters that advertise the benefit of fiber, fat and the latest craze, molecular hydrogen.

Gatorade, created at the University of Florida College of Medicine in

1965, is a balance of carbohydrates and electrolytes. It was designed to aid in fluid replacement for the Florida Gators football players. Gatorade beverage is meant for athletes who are exercising in extreme conditions, like marathons and triathlons, or in the instance of the Gators, playing football in the sweltering Florida heat. It's not meant for your average Jane or Joe spending an hour on the treadmill at the gym. It's unlikely the body's stores of these minerals are depleted during a typical training session. And since all of these sports drinks contain about 60 to 100 calories per eight-ounce serving, you would be the gerbil on the wheel chasing your calorie-laden tail.

**Thousands have lived without love, not one without water.**

–H. AUDEN, ENGLISH-AMERICAN POET

Except for zero-calorie flavored waters and diet drinks, just about all other manufactured, nonalcoholic beverages rely heavily on three significant substances: sugar, caffeine, and surprisingly, salt. The body doesn't need sugar or caffeine. They're not necessary for our survival. We only need water—clean water. Drinking other beverages may have unwanted side effects. In excess, caffeine can trigger excitation, insomnia, and headaches. In excess, sugar can quickly put on unwanted pounds leading to other health risks.

Remember, the body doesn't need sugar to stay alive, but it does need water.

The sugar found in these sweetened beverages not only adds empty calories but has a detrimental effect on the brain. Children are most at risk as their brains are in the developmental stages.

Coca-Cola spends approximately $3.8 billion a year on advertising. Divided by a world population of 7.5 billion, this works out to about fifty cents for every person on earth. It makes sense, because annually per capita, the world population spends almost three dollars each on Coca-Cola products.

68

The sugar in soda beverages light up the pleasure centers of the brain in the same manner as heroin. The brain produces dopamine, a neurotransmitter, and it's that happy hormone that lights up the brain like fireworks on the Fourth of July, making the experience of consuming sugary drinks pleasurable for our brain.

Although these beverages have been deemed safe to drink occasionally, they add no value to your nutritional needs. As Paracelsus said anything could become poisonous to the body, depending on the quantity. With sugary beverages, it doesn't take much for these beverages to become a detriment to your overall health.

*A 330ml can of Coca Cola contains so much sugar, your body should vomit— but the phosphoric acid "cuts the flavor, helping you keep the liquid down.*
—WADE MEREDITH, HEALTH WRITER, THE TELEGRAPH, JULY 30, 2015

When it comes to added sugar consumption, the American Heart Association recommends no more than six teaspoons for women and nine teaspoons for men per day. On average, Americans consume approximately seventeen teaspoons daily, which added up amounts to fifty-seven pounds of added sugar consumed each year, per person. Making it even more confusing, most soft drinks report sugar content in grams instead of teaspoons. About four grams equals one teaspoon of sugar. Most people would be shocked by the amount of sugar they unknowingly consume.

It becomes alarming when you do the math and see how it relates to soft drinks. Consider a woman who has a regular diet of about 2,000 calories to maintain a healthy weight. One day she decides to drink a twenty-ounce sugary soft drink. Every day after that for a year, she repeats this daily habit. Changing no other exercise, lifestyle, or diet routines, after the year, she would have gained approximately twenty-four pounds.

Added sugar consumption through your beverage choice can easily be an unconscious slip that develops into an unhealthy dietary habit. The seemingly harmless act of adding one soft drink a day could prove to be detrimental to your long-term health.

## WHAT WATER DOES FOR YOUR BODY

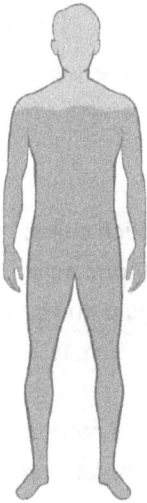

**Breaks down food for nutrient absorption**

**Flushes Body's waste, urine**

**Lubricates joints**

**Keeps mucosal membranes moist**

**Supports cell growth**

**Supports brain to produce hormones and neurotransmitters**

**Regulates body temperature (sweating and respiration)**

**Acts as a shock absorber for brain and spinal cord function**

**Help deliver oxygen to the cells of the body**

## BOTTOMS UP

Roughly 30 percent of American adults are teetotalers—those who abstain from alcoholic beverages altogether. Another 30 percent of the population consumes less than one alcoholic drink per week. Meaning a large portion of the population don't consume much alcohol at all.

> *I envy people who drink. At least they have something to blame everything on.*
> —OSCAR LEVANT, AMERICAN PIANIST AND COMPOSER

Heavy alcohol use is linked to an increased likelihood of using drugs. Heavy consumption can also lead to liver disease, kill brain cells, and contribute to other chronic diseases. Another good reason to refrain is that alcohol may trigger past emotional traumas and contribute to depression or anxiety.

With approximately 60 percent of the population mostly abstaining, producing beer, wine, and spirits might seem like a meager way to make a living. But there you would be wrong.

> **One reason I don't drink is that I want to know when I am having a good time.**
> —NANCY ASTOR, SOCIALITE, AND WIFE OF WALDORF ASTOR

The majority of the sales of alcoholic beverages come from about 40 percent of the population.[19] Ten percent of American adults consume between ten and a whopping seventy-five drinks per week. As an example, seventy-five alcoholic drinks could break down into roughly one of the following: four and a half bottles of Jack Daniels, eighteen bottles of wine, or three twenty-four-can cases of beer.

The top 10 percent of drinkers account for well over half the alcohol consumed in any given year.[20]

> **Of all the vices, drinking is the most incompatible with greatness.**
> —SIR WALTER SCOTT, SCOTTISH HISTORICAL NOVELIST

But how much is too much?

It depends on body weight and composition. It's generally believed that one drink per hour, along with one glass of water, would allow the body to maintain a reasonable blood alcohol level. An average man drinking a twelve-ounce beer would have an approximate blood alcohol content (BAC) of 0.025 percent, well below the legal limit of 0.08 percent BAC. Of course, the blood alcohol content for a petite woman would be much higher.

As an example, for a healthy, average-size male, it would take his liver about one hour to metabolize a little less than one standard drink. There's no way to speed this process up, but eating before and after drinking can slow the absorption of alcohol into the system.

Alcohol is often a way to get the party started and to help people relax. A drink can improve our mood, elevate our self-confidence, lower anxiety, and take the edge off. But there's a limit: too much alcohol and our elevated mood can turn for the worse, leaving us with feelings of sadness, guilt and regret.

A BAC of 0.09 percent puts your BAC over the legal limit. Depending on your size, that could be less than one drink per hour. Keep drinking and your attention span shortens, your vision blurs, motor skills and balance are impaired, and your judgment is compromised. Keep drinking more and you could be heading to severe problems with amnesia, loss of consciousness, vomiting, respiratory depression, and potentially death.

Chronic alcohol abuse may be the cause of other issues. Some people drink alcohol in an attempt to cope with depression or anxieties. Self-medicating with alcohol may lead to a physical dependency or a gateway to other damaging drugs or behaviors.

> *For women, low-risk drinking is no more than three drinks on any single day and no more than seven drinks per week. For men, it is defined as no more than four drinks on any single day and no more than fourteen drinks per week.*
> —NATIONAL INSTITUTE ON ALCOHOL ABUSE AND ALCOHOLISM'S DEFINITION OF LOW RISK DRINKING FOR DEVELOPING ALCOHOL USE DISORDER

From a bottle of beer to a glass of wine or a shot of tequila, most alcohol contains calories. A 12-ounce container of beer can easily range from about 100 calories to over 350 calories, depending on whether it's a light beer or a deep ale. With the later, it wouldn't take long to blow your diet by having a few beers. Fat stores from increased alcohol consumption tend to accumulate in the abdominal area, thus the creation of the beer belly.

> **If you ever reach total enlightenment while drinking beer,**
> **I bet it makes beer shoot out your nose.**
> —JACK HANDY, AMERICAN HUMORIST

Millions of American adults regularly enjoy a glass of wine, a beer, or a cocktail responsibly. Establish your drinking goal, and don't deviate from your plan. Base your alcohol consumption on what is best for your long-term health and lifestyle.

When it comes to alcohol, Paracelsus couldn't be more right—there comes a point when too much becomes poisonous.

> **I'm very serious about no alcohol, no drugs. Life is too beautiful.**
> —JIM CAREY, COMEDIAN

In the next chapter, how three simple rules can change your relationship with food and your long-term health.

---

## CHAPTER SUMMARY

☑ Upon rising, drink one to two glasses of water to rehydrate your brain and body.

☑ Drink the proper amount of water for your needs. Be aware not to drink so much you blow out your electrolyte balance, but drink a steady amount so your kidneys can adequately process all fluids.

☑ Know your alcohol limits and stick to them.

## CHAPTER SIX

# How "Health" Food Landed Me in The Hospital

*The food you eat can be either the safest and most powerful form of medicine or the slowest form of poison.*
—ANN WIGMORE, THE ANN WIGMORE NATURAL HEALTH INSTITUTE

## LIFE-CHALLENGING EVENT NUMBER TWO

It was the third day of our annual sojourn to Maui, one of my favorite surfing destinations. It was late in the evening when I felt the first sharp abdominal pain. It was a severe cramping sensation that sent me flying to the nearest toilet. I succumbed to the immediate urge to poo, and when I finished, I turned to flush. I stood there startled. There was blood in the toilet. What? I was confused. The pain wasn't horrible, but there was a lot of blood. A few minutes later, more blood.

It was late in the evening—too late to make a fuss. Anyway, where would I go? I was on an island, my options were limited, and the area urgent care clinic had closed. Since the pain wasn't horrible, I thought maybe it was a temporary situation and would clear up by morning. I decided a sleeping pill would be the easiest way to get to sleep and put the worries out of my head.

The effects of the sleeping pill wore off around 4:00 am. The pain was back, only worse, and with more blood. I decided this was serious. I woke my husband, Jack, and told him I was feeling pretty bad and I thought I should go to the hospital. He was having a hard time waking up. I told him to take his time, that I was okay—I lied. He got it together as fast as he could, and we headed across the island to Maui Memorial Medical Center in Wailuku.

It was still dark when we arrived. We were the only ones in the emergency room, and I was quickly shuffled into an exam room. The internal medicine doctor on call was phoned, and he showed up about a half-hour later dressed in flip-flops, board shorts, and a T-shirt. A big swell was coming in, and he was headed to catch some early morning waves when he got the call. (Only in Hawaii, right?)

By his looks, I guessed he was a native Hawaiian—the tussle of unruly black hair, creamy beige skin, and mixed ethnicity of Asian descendants. I was thrilled he was a surfer, as I was too, and before much else, I asked him about the surf conditions on the part of the island he surfed. He was accommodating, charming and yet direct as he turned the questions back to my health. Was I pregnant? Had I experienced a blunt trauma to my abdomen? Eaten any raw or questionable foods? No, no, and no. I had done nothing unusual. I couldn't imagine why this was happening.

I was quickly admitted, tests were ordered, and blood was crossmatched for possible transfusion depending on how much more blood I lost. I was scared. This was out of left field, and I seemed to be getting worse. The blood kept coming. I felt I was fading and getting weaker.

Across the way, a visitor played the ukulele for a family member. The sound of people walking in flip-flops resonated from the hall. My roommate, an elderly woman, announced to the nurse she had to "chee, chee." I found out later that was Hawaiian slang for having to pee. Other only-in-Hawaii things popped up in the hospital: coconut Jell-O, mango

75

fruit juice, Hawaiian-print hospital gowns, doctors in Hawaiian-print shirts, and flowers that smelled and looked exotic. I wound up spending three days in Maui Memorial Medical Center. If you're ever sick in Maui, I highly recommend the experience.

On the third day, I was discharged from the hospital hours before my flight back to Los Angeles. The internal bleeding had stopped, but the doctors at Maui Memorial never determined the cause. After all the specialists, scans, tests, and a colonoscopy, they confirmed only that my intestinal tract had somehow failed, and blood was leaking from my bloodstream through my intestinal wall and into my colon. I was instructed to follow up with my regular doctors in Los Angeles, and I did.

My doctor in Los Angeles is a slender man with kind blue eyes. As a Sikh, he wears a distinctive white turban. Over the years, I have seen his wiry, long beard turn from ashen brown to dusty white. He has been my trusted advisor and has pulled me out of a few healthcare scares.

He practices integrative medicine, blending a holistic approach to both Eastern and Western medical traditions. An office visit often includes muscle testing, naturopathy, acupuncture, vitamins, and minerals, to give patients the best in all forms of healthcare. As far as my case went, he was baffled. There didn't seem to be any clear-cut cause for why my system failed. More tests were ordered and reviewed, and nothing jumped out. As a last resort, we talked about food testing.

The new test might provide a diagnostic tool to identify and measure autoimmune reactivity that could affect multiple areas of my body's tissues. These types of tests were relatively new to the market, and I was excited to see what might turn up.

A blood draw was performed and shipped off to the lab. Within a couple of days, I was sitting back with my doctor. The results were shocking. Literally, they were off the charts.

Among the substances tested were gluten proteins, which are found in grains like wheat, rye, spelt, and barley. Of the gluten-containing grains, wheat is the most commonly consumed through bread, pasta, pastries, and other yummy dough products. When flour is mixed with water, it's the gluten that gives the dough its elasticity and bread the ability to rise when baked. Peel apart a crusty loaf of freshly baked bread, and you'll see air pockets. Gluten is the sticky substance that traps the air and forms these bubbles, making the texture of bread to die for (literally, as it would turn out in my case.)

The gluten testing scale went from 0 to 20, and my score—47—was off the chart. The cause of my internal bleeding may or may not have been associated with the gluten allergy—which has remained a mystery. But the news of how far off the scale I was caused concern and could have been the source of other issues I faced.

Years earlier, I don't remember exactly when it was, I started feeling a deep malaise. It had become constant, like I was getting the flu. I ached all over, felt weak, and had headaches that made me want to curl up in a ball on the couch. I felt I was dragging myself through life. Added to it, I had digestive problems that years before had been diagnosed as irritable bowel syndrome.

During all that time, I felt lost. It didn't seem that anything I did helped. It was a lot to face each day. The diagnosis of a severe gluten allergy finally made some sense. I thought, it might be the answer to the question of why I felt so lousy all the time.

For years, my morning ritual was a small bowl of shredded wheat, topped with slivered almonds and blueberries, all floating in a pool of almond milk. It's pretty delicious, "healthy" stuff. Right? Wrong. It all made sense now: my morning ritual was the worst thing I could have been doing. After the diagnosis, I never consciously ate a gluten product again. It wasn't easy, as so many products have wheat in them. Who knew soy sauce contains wheat? That red licorice is full of wheat? As well as many soups, salad dressings, and other products that use flour as thickeners?

It took some changes, but after a couple of months of being gluten-free I felt better than I had in years. I asked my husband in disbelief, "Is this what normal feels like?" I wanted to cry thinking of all the time I had spent feeling miserable. I couldn't believe I could feel so good from something as simple as giving up flour.

*"Let food by thy medicine and medicine be thy food."* This profound quote is most often ascribed to Hippocrates, an ancient Greek philosopher dating back to 400 BC. Although there's no evidence Hippocrates said it, the concept of food as your medicine resonates and emphasizes the importance of our food choices in our quest for health.

Having a gluten allergy, then unknowingly eating it for years, is like eating small amounts of poison. The result of this daily poisoning created what's known as leaky gut syndrome. This is not some new-fangled, made-up disease. It's more common than you might imagine, but not until recent years did medicine have the ability to test for it.

The blood test I mentioned earlier tests to see if gluten proteins are floating around in your blood. They're not supposed to be there. The wall of your intestine is supposed to prevent the foreign undigested gluten protein matter from entering your bloodstream. The fact that these proteins had migrated into my blood, and in record numbers, meant my intestinal wall failed to do its job. If you're celiac or have a wheat sensitivity, the wheat acts as an irritant to the lining of your intestinal tract and over time can create gaps in the lining.

This is a problem, as it allows the gluten protein molecules to migrate into the bloodstream. The body reacts to these proteins as foreign matter and sets off the body's immune response. Inflammation, digestive problems, headaches, joint pain, and a plethora of other discomforts ensue. It never occurred to me—this could all be from pizza night with the hubby. If I only knew the damage I was doing.

It's hard for me to look back and pinpoint when I started to feel so bad. It doesn't matter when. Today, knowing the source of my health problems gave me a solid answer to why I felt terrible, and the strategy to change my eating habits forever.

## YUMMY, FOOD FOR MY TUMMY... AND ALL THE BUGS INSIDE ME

Billions of years ago, single-cell organisms were the earliest living things. They just floated around taking in food through their cell walls. Fast-forward billions of years, digestive pathways and stomachs evolved, then jaws and teeth. For humans, our brains got bigger, and our nutritional needs increased. Our senses developed to seek out a more abundant variety of nutrients to feed our system, our bigger brains, and our evolutionary needs.

Humans were able to evolve more efficiently when we found that fire cooks our food, especially meat, ridding it of dangerous pathogens and making it palatable. Cooking also breaks down plant foods' cell walls. For example, dried beans, cooking helps start the long digestive process and aids in our ability to extract certain nutrients. Cooking meant we could feed our brains more efficiently, allowing more time to develop cognitive abilities rather than spending our time foraging for food. No other species on the planet cooks their food. That alone may have been the fork in the evolutionary road that helped us develop complex big brains.

*Homo erectus's* evolving bigger brain meant his caloric intake had to increase to accommodate the nutritional needs of his brain. Our modern brain takes up 20 percent of our energy needs, but our brain is only about 2 percent of our body mass, making it an energy hog.

The brain has other surprising needs. The brain connects to the gut by the vagus nerve. The vagus nerve is the longest and most complicated nerve of the body running from the brain through the face and chest into the abdomen. The trillions of microbes that make up your gut microbiome create chemicals that travel up the vagus nerve and affect how your brain works. Like a phone system, these chemicals can call up the brain to eat less and curb cravings. They can affect mood, fear, anxiety, inflammation, and pain, and they have a whole host of other biological effects. In other words, the gut microbiome and its bacteria can control your moods, pain, and so much more. The complexity of the gut microbiome and its specific effects on the body has fast become the topic of major research and may provide further ground-breaking discoveries.

In one such study, feeding mice a probiotic that altered their gut microbiome helped reduce the amount of stress hormone in their blood. However, if their vagus nerve was cut severing the connection between the brain and the gut, the probiotic had no effect. Proving the microbes in the gut have huge effects on the brain.[21]

For example, some of these microbes make short-chain fatty acids (SCFA) from the fiber we eat. These SCFAs can affect the brain in several ways, such as reducing appetite and cravings. Serotonin, most of which is produced by the gut, creates feelings of happiness, while gamma-aminobutyric acid (GABA) aids in controlling feelings of fear and anxiety.

## YOUR SECOND BRAIN: YOUR GUT MICROBIOME

Your gut's microbiome consists of tens of trillions of microorganisms that weigh approximately three to four pounds, and include at least a thousand different species of known bacteria. These bacteria are hungry, but these little bugs are dependent on you to feed them. What you put in your pie hole filters down to what's on the menu for these microbes to eat.

*Biology will relate every human gene to the genes of other animals and bacteria, to this great chain of being.*
—WALTER GILBERT, AMERICAN BIOCHEMIST, NOBEL LAUREATE

This natural requirement to feed our gut microbes is evident even with newborns. For all of humankind, a mother's breast milk has been the ideal nourishment to help babies grow. What's surprising is approximately 10 percent of the breast milk is completely indigestible by babies and of seemingly no nutritional value. Made up of complex sugars called oligosaccharides, babies lack the enzymes to digest or absorb this material. It seems evolution would have eliminated this biomolecule if it was of no use to the child's growth or development. So, why is it there?

Evolution was involved, but not for the baby per se. It's to feed what's inside the baby—the baby's microbiome. Evolutionary strategy allowed mothers' bodies to produce the food required for the development of the baby's gut microbiome. These oligosaccharides nurture the growth of good bacteria that builds up the baby's immune system and helps to protect it from infections.[22]

Our gut microbiome plays a variety of crucial roles in how we absorb and use nutrients from our foods. Remember, the gut microbiome eats whatever we eat. Then the bacteria's waste products are utilized by our own body to help synthesize our nutrients—all the more reason that the variety and health of these microbes are so important for a healthy immune system and for disease prevention. Your microbiome may also affect the central nervous system and brain function, as well as play a large part in weight gain, mood, diabetes, heart disease, and the risk of cancer.[23]

For example, scientists analyzed stool samples from 1,300 sets of twins to understand what types of bacteria lived in their guts. That analysis gave them two results.

First, a certain proportion of gut bacteria seems to be inherited.

Second, people with less bacterial diversity in their gut had a higher percentage of visceral fat. Obesity somehow correlates with having less diverse gut bacteria.[24]

Two gut bacteria, *Bacteroidetes* and *Firmicutes*, were found to be possibly linked with weight gain. In an experiment, lean and obese mice had their gut microbiomes manipulated. The obese mice harvested more energy or calories from their foods, and this adversely affected their metabolism, making them obese. The effect could then be transmitted by colonizing the lean mouse's gut with the microbiome of the obese mouse. That slowed the lean mouse's metabolism and created weight gain similar to that of the obese mouse. The results indicated that the gut microbiome has an impact on metabolic function and weight gain.[25]

There have also been studies of the gut microbiome and how it's involved in chronic pain. In one such study, approximately nineteen different bacteria were found in the microbiome of patients with fibromyalgia. Emmanuel Gonzalez of the Canadian Center for Computational Genomics at McGill University's Department of Human Genetics states:

"We sorted through large amounts of data, identifying nineteen species that were either increased or decreased in individuals with fibromyalgia. By using machine learning, our computer was able to make a diagnosis of fibromyalgia, based only on the composition of the microbiome, with an accuracy of 87 percent. As we build on this first discovery with more research, we hope to improve upon this accuracy, potentially creating a step-change in diagnosis."[26]

Fibromyalgia and several other chronic diseases are being analyzed from the perspective of our gut bacteria. There is hope, and early work shows promise, in this new area of research to identify chronic diseases and characterize possible links.

In 1826, Anthelme Brillat-Savarin said, "Tell me what you eat, and I will tell you what you are." Meaning if you eat well, you will be well. The nutritional content of what you eat affects how well your body repairs the billions of cells it replaces daily. When we consider the critical role of the gut microbiome, maybe the interpretation would be, "You are what your gut microbiome eats."

## CHOW DOWN

There are only two things your body can do with the calories in the foods you eat: use them as energy or turn them into fat. That's pretty much it.

Your first energy requirements are to maintain your basal metabolic rate (BMR). The BMR is the number of calories required to keep your body functioning at complete rest. These are the calories needed for all your bodily functions like breathing, digestion, circulation, and keeping your heart pumping.

Your second energy requirements are those calories needed for your daily movements. Whether it's standing, walking, running a marathon or just sitting upright on the couch, you need calories to provide the energy for these activities.

After that, any additional unused calories are stored as fat. So, if you eat more calories than what you use, then the only option the body has is to store them as fat. But it's also not that simple. What the body can use is dependent on your metabolism, genetics, and as we have learned, the health of your gut microbiome.

Your BMR can vary depending on your level of fitness. As explained, even without doing anything, your heart continues beating, blood still flows, kidneys keep making urine, digestion is still going on, and, of course, you're still breathing. However, the more muscle mass you have, the more calories your body needs to sit around and do nothing. The cells of the body, like the muscles, need a certain number of calories to be maintained, repaired and replaced when needed. So, the fitter you are, the bigger your engine, and the higher your caloric needs for your BMR.

Jack LaLanne, "Godfather of Fitness," pioneered the fitness industry through his popular morning television show, *The Jack LaLanne Show*. It was the longest-running exercise show, airing in 1953 and running until 1985. LaLanne opened dozens of gyms, published books, designed exercise equipment, produced vitamin supplements, and asserted processed food was to blame for many health problems.

LaLanne summed up his view of fitness and nutrition:

"Dying is easy. Living is a pain in the butt. It's like an athletic event. You've got to train for it. You've got to eat right. You've got to exercise. Your health account, your bank account, they're the same thing. The more you put in, the more you can take out. Exercise is king, and nutrition is queen: together, you have a kingdom."[27]

LaLanne said his two simple rules of nutrition are, "If man made it, don't eat it." and "if it tastes good, spit it out."[28]

People in the 1950s were trim and fit and weighed on average twenty-five pounds less than people today. In 1960, the weight of the average American man, forty to sixty years old, was one hundred sixty-six pounds. Today that number is over two hundred pounds—an increase of thirty-four pounds or over a 20 percent weight increase in one generation.[29]

Now, 160 million Americans, nearly half the population, are either obese or overweight. Almost 75 percent of American men and more than 60 percent of women are obese or overweight.[30]

A recent post published on the website of the American Medical

Association reports the obesity rate is at 40 percent. This is up dramatically since the period between 2005 and 2012, when the obesity rate was about 35 percent, and an apocalyptic rise since 1980 when the obesity rate was a mere 15 percent. That's a significant change in only a few decades.

Approximately eight hundred thousand people died in 2019 from heart attacks or strokes. That's the equivalent of four 747 jumbo jets filled with people crashing into the ground every day for a year. Just let that sink in.

In March 2019, after two Boeing 737 MAX 8 series aircraft crashed, one involving Ethiopian Airlines and the other Lion Air in Indonesia, the Federal Aviation Administration (FAA) grounded all of the Boeing series planes in the United States, and thirty countries around the world did the same. After these two crashes, over three hundred aircraft remained grounded until a thorough investigation could be completed. When it comes to our health and dying of obesity-related problems, as a nation, and as the world, what have we done to collectively turn the tide?

Since the trim waistlines of the 1950s, we've been bombarded with diet strategies. Diets touting low carbs versus low fat, but nothing has worked. Our waistlines are ever-expanding, and obesity rates are projected to rise to 50 percent by 2030.

In 1958, 1.6 million people were diagnosed with diabetes.[31] Today, The Centers for Disease Control and Prevention report more than 100 million Americans, or 30 percent of the population, have diabetes or are prediabetic. This growing number has added an enormous burden to the health care system.[32] With an estimated average lifetime cost of $85,200 per person with diabetes, the health care system may not be sustainable.[33]

With the prognosis getting worse, what is the diagnosis? What could be the cure to avert this trend? To find a solution, we need to go back in history to the beginning of the war between fat and sugar.

# THE WAR BETWEEN FAT AND SUGAR

In May 1945, Adolf Hitler committed suicide. Within a week Allied forces accepted Germany's surrender, and the war in Asia officially ended on September 2, 1945, with the surrender of Japan. World War II was over, and men were coming home to their sweethearts, getting married, starting families, and enjoying the good life.

During the war, soldiers were issued C-rations. C-rations are prepared, canned, and ready-to-eat combat food rations. Included in the C-rations were packs of unfiltered cigarettes. In the stressful environment of war, many took to smoking the readily available cigarettes and continued the habit once they got back home. Women also lit up, and by the 1960s an estimated 42 percent of Americans regularly smoked.

It's been widely documented that for these postwar Americans, the "good life" meant smoking, drinking, and eating an unhealthy diet. Beginning in the 1950s, heart disease and strokes were on an epic rise, and people were dying. On a September afternoon in 1955, the situation caught national attention when President Dwight D. Eisenhower, age sixty-four, complained of indigestion. Within twenty-four hours, he was admitted to Fitzsimons Army Hospital under the care of the top cardiologist. The man who had been a five-star general and Supreme Allied Commander in Europe spent the next six weeks in the hospital.[34] The American public was updated daily, and heart disease became public enemy number one.

In this era before the invention of statins, the cholesterol-lowering medication, something had to be done. Someone had to make sense of all this.

Ancel Keys was an American physiologist. He studied the influence of diet on health, which led him to the hypothesis that dietary fat was the culprit in the increased rate of heart disease Americans were experiencing. The fat in the diet adversely affected serum cholesterol levels, and he set out to prove his hypothesis with his controversial "Seven County Study" published in 1958.

The countries in the study where fat consumption was highest had higher rates of heart disease, leading Keys to conclude it was the dietary fat that caused heart disease. Keys was among the first to examine diet and disease, collaborating with scientists worldwide.

In later years, Keys has faced controversy, including accusations he cherry-picked countries to support his hypothesis. That only seven countries were considered out of the twenty-two countries examined led to inaccuracies. Skeptics claim Norway and Holland were excluded because they had low rates of heart disease but consumed loads of fat. Chile was excluded because they ate little fat but had high rates of heart disease. Whether the data was flawed or not, the information presented in Keys' study gained massive media attention. His research influenced national dietary guidelines that encouraged the American public to adopt a low-fat diet.

Yet our fat consumption over the decades has skyrocketed, from 147 grams in 1970 to 190 in 2010, and climbing. Statistics show Americans never went on the low-fat diet recommended by Ancel Keys, and have just gotten bigger and bigger.

The second controversy in the Keys study comes from his relationship with the sugar producers.

In 1954, the trade group called the Sugar Research Foundation (SRF), known today as the Sugar Association, may have influenced Ancel Keys to discount sugar as a dietary factor in his studies. That year the president of the SRF gave a speech claiming if Americans adopted a lower-fat diet, they would need to replace the taste of fat with something else. This was a unique business opportunity—to replace the fat with sugar in manufactured food products to make their taste more appealing.[35]

Before the twentieth century, Americans consumed about two pounds of sugar a year. Today the average American consumes over one hundred fifty-two pounds of sugar each year, which equates to six cups of sugar a week and roughly forty teaspoons a day. This represents a shocking 76 percent increase in sugar consumption. The American Heart Association recommends adult women consume less than six teaspoons of sugar per day, and adult men consume less than nine teaspoons. Today, processed sugar and other sugar derivatives are added to three out of four food products found on grocery store shelves.[36]

Here's the rub.

The book *Pure, White and Deadly*, published in 1972 by Professor John Yudkin, a British physiologist and nutritionist, was the culmination of his years of research and focus on treating the overweight and on the harmful effects of excessive sugar consumption.

As early as 1958, Yudkin showed most patients' weight could be controlled by restricting dietary carbohydrates and sugar. He published an easy guide to weight loss in the book titled *This Slimming Business* in 1958, which reached its fourth edition in 1974. Yudkin found sugar consumption to have the closest relationship to coronary deaths over any single dietary factor. That included fat, which had been highly publicized as the culprit during the same time frame.

Yudkin's ideas were gaining traction with the American public as well as sparking deep concern from the Sugar Research Association and Ancel Keys. They were none too happy about having the finger pointed at sugar.

Yudkin threw down the gauntlet. The end of the first chapter of *Pure, White and Deadly* begins, "I hope that when you have read this book I shall have convinced you that sugar is really dangerous."

The war had begun.

Yudkin's book and research didn't go over well with the sugar industry or the food manufacturers who adopted the strategy of added sugar to enhance the taste of their products. It was one man, Yudkin, against the giants in the food industry, and Yudkin lost. The food industry and sugar launched an all-out attack with the help of their key player, Ancel Keys who wrote:

"It is clear that Yudkin has no theoretical basis or experimental evidence to support his claim for a major influence of dietary sucrose in the etiology of Coronary Heart Disease (CHD); his claim that men who have CHD are excessive sugar eaters is nowhere confirmed but is disproved by many studies superior in methodology and/or magnitude to his own; and his "evidence" from population statistics and time trends will not bear up under the most elementary critical examination. But the propaganda keeps on reverberating ..."[37]

Personal smears and dismissive language used by Ancel Keys against John Yudkin were overwhelming, and the mild-mannered Yudkin was ill-equipped in the art of political combat. By the time of Yudkin's death in 1995, his warnings on the devastation of sugar had been long lost in the milieu of Keys's attacks. For a time, Yudkin's theory about sugar was taken seriously but was buried—not by opposing scientific fact, but by a smear campaign, and the influence of a powerful few.

In the 1970s, the Sugar Association, worried about its public image, targeted newspaper ads to a new demographic of women who were concerned about their weight. The campaign, "Sugar can be the willpower you need to under-eat," spoke to the heart of these women. The following year, the executives from the Sugar Association received the Oscar of the PR world, the Silver Anvil Award, for their excellence in "the forging of public opinion." This and successfully swaying the FDA to change its ruling on the adverse effects of sugar put sugar in the clear. Fat and the birth of the low-fat craze gained the traction the sugar industry was looking for. Now sugar is off the hook, and the food industry is on board with creating new food products to market.

## SOME COMMON NAMES FOR SUGAR

| | | | |
|---|---|---|---|
| Agave | Coconut | High fructose | Maple syrup |
| Barley malt | sugar | corn syrup | Palm sugar |
| Beet sugar | Corn syrup | Fruit sugar | Raw sugar |
| Blackstrap | Corn | Galactose | Rice syrup |
| molasses | sweetener | Glucose | Saccharose |
| Brown sugar | Demerara | Grape juice | Sorghum |
| Brown rice | sugar | concentrate | Sucrose |
| syrup | Date sugar | Grape sugar | Sugar |
| Cane juice | Dextrin | Honey Invert | Treacle |
| Cane sugar | Dextrose | sugar | Turbinado |
| Caramel | Diastatic malt | Lactose | Sugar |
| Carob syrup | Evaporated | Maltodextrin | Xylose |
| | cane juice | Maltose | |

**FOUR MOST COMMON USED SWEETENERS**
**CORN SYRUP, HIGH-FRUCTOSE CORN SYRUP,**
**FRUIT JUICE CONCENTRATES, CANE SUGARS**

## SUGAR—HOW SWEET IT ISN'T

Processed white sugar and most other sugars, including natural sugars like honey, have little to no nutritional value and are mostly empty calories. The body has no biological or functional need for sugar of any kind. You could eliminate sugar from your diet as the body has no fundamental need for it. Most likely, your body would be better off without it, as sugar does have damaging effects on the body.

There are at least fifty-six different names for sugar. Honey, a natural sugar, contains fructose, glucose, maltose, and sucrose. It has no fiber, fat, or protein. Processed white sugar is higher on the glycemic index, meaning it raises blood sugar levels more quickly. Natural honey does contain certain amounts of nutrients like vitamins and minerals, but nothing the body can't get from other foods. Honey, although natural, is still a form of sugar, and can affect your blood glucose level in much the same way as regular table sugar. In the brain, high amounts of sugar impair both our cognitive skills and our cravings or self-control. Sugar can stimulate a drug-like effect and has been known to be more addictive than heroin, which we touched on in our soda discussion. The reward centers of the brain fire up, telling us sugar is delicious. The only benefit sugar may have is that it fires the brain in pleasure, and our taste buds read it as irresistible. Although pleasurable, most sugars are a nutritionally wasteland.

We may be genetically predisposed to hunt out sweet things. This predisposition was a way to signal our early ancestors when fruit was ripe to eat—by the sweetness. But our early ancestors only had things like fruits that contained natural sugars to choose from, not foods laden with processed sugars. If you have hankering for something sweet, it would be better to choose whole-foods high in natural sugar, like fruits, instead of processed sugars or manufactured foods with added sugars. There's room in the diet for a little sweetness but the key is to limit all sugars both in quantity and quality.

Your body can only metabolize so much sugar at one time, including natural sugars. When you eat an abundance of sugar, your pancreas produces the hormone insulin. Insulin acts like a key to unlock the cell so glucose (sugar) can enter and the cell can use it for energy. Bombarding the bloodstream with large amounts of sugar taxes this fragile system. The body stores excess sugar as fat in the liver and elsewhere, and is one of the causes of fatty liver disease.

Sugar is also known to cause teeth to decay and lead to cavities. It's the oxidative damage that causes the tooth decay. The same oxidative damage doesn't end with just the mouth—it can damage the blood vessels and fragile capillaries in the same way, leading to the hardening of the arteries and possibly organ damage.

The journey to removing sugar from your diet or lowering your sugar intake will take effort. The University of North Carolina conducted a detailed survey of packaged food in most grocery stores and found 60 percent of foods contain added sugar. Sugar was added to the product presumably as a flavor enhancer. High-fructose corn syrup, one of the different names for sugar, is much sweeter than regular cane sugar and less expensive. It also acts as a preservative so packaged goods will last longer on the shelf, making added high-fructose corn syrup a win-win for the food industry.

## DOES FAT MAKE YOU THIN?

Your body needs fat. You would die if you didn't eat some fat. Fat, and specifically the essential fatty acids, the scientific term for fats the body has to get from the diet, help us in many ways and are crucial to life. They store energy, provide insulation, and protect our organs as well as aid in the biochemical process of absorbing fat-soluble vitamins. They help proteins do their job, support immune functions and reproduction, and aid in other aspects of metabolism.

All good—but here's the rub. We have two problems: many of us eat too much fat and more importantly, the wrong kinds of fat.

Fat has nine calories per gram, making it calorically denser than carbohydrates or protein. Per gram, fat has more than twice as many calories as carbohydrates or proteins.

As an example, the caloric content in two tablespoons of olive oil is about the same as that in ten cups of broccoli. I doubt most people could eat ten cups of broccoli at a meal, but it's easy to have a couple of tablespoons of olive oil. Fat may make foods more satisfying, but fats don't have the bulk of something like broccoli and fat alone isn't filling to the stomach. There's no bulk leaving us hungry for more.

By comparison, an avocado is about 77 percent fat, making them higher in fat than most animal foods. And an average avocado has about the

same calorie content as two tablespoons of olive oil or ten cups of broccoli. One avocado just can't compare in bulk to ten cups of broccoli, but
avocados are delicious and offer other nutritional benefits.

So, what's the problem?

The body processes fat differently than carbs or protein. For energy,
your body will burn carbs and even protein before it burns fat. If the fat
you've consumed is not used as energy then it is stored as fat gain in
the body. Making consuming fat a balance between how much fat is too
much and when your fat intake contributes to your body's fat stores.

We also eat the wrong kinds of fats.

Saturated fats are solid at room temperature, unlike unsaturated fats,
which are liquid at room temperature. Sources of saturated fats include:
red meat, some pork and chicken products, and dairy products. These
fats may increase your risk of heart disease, type 2 diabetes and other
chronic illnesses, whereas unsaturated fats, mostly found in oils from
nuts, seeds, olives, and vegetables, are less likely to cause adverse
health effects.

Or are they?

The widely held belief is that unsaturated fats are good for your overall
health and have even been named heart healthy. Although more definitive
research is needed, certain cooking oils go through a heavy manufacturing process that includes high heat, chemicals, bleaching and more. This
heavy processing changes the chemical make-up of the oils creating free
radicals. Free radicals may cause cellular damage, in particular damage
to the arteries, and are linked to a host of other health concerns.

A good rule of thumb is nature does not make bad fats—heavy manufacturing does. Go for expeller-pressed oils, like olive oils or minimally

processed oils, even butter, instead of heavily manufactured ones like corn, canola, soybean, or other vegetable oils.

## FOOD PORN

The number of meals you eat in a day depends on your energy needs. Most of us eat breakfast, lunch, and dinner, but there is no biological reason why, and the scheduling may be more of a comfort in predictability than necessity.

In the 1920s, the government promoted breakfast as a way for workers to have the energy to make it through the day. Today, we receive food messages from our environment—the look and smell of food fires our brain and signal us to eat up.

Take donuts, for example. Donuts can be a delightfully delicious treat. They even look delicious—a frosted cacophony of flavors mixing fat, sugar, and yumminess. The aroma of donuts entices you to stop and enjoy. But what if you're driving, sealed in your air-conditioned car, unable to smell or even see the soldier-straight rows of frosted perfection? That's okay, Krispy Kreme has you covered. Employees flip the switch on a large, neon red, "Hot Now" sign that visually lets you know fresh donuts are available. You don't need to smell them. Just see the red, neon light, and like Pavlov's dog trained to respond, your brain goes into donut mode.

Krispy Kreme's hope is once you have tasted their fresh, hot-from-the-fryer donuts, you'll be hooked and become a loyal fan. So faithful you'll download their Hot Light app. No matter where you are, you can find the nearest Krispy Kreme, and be notified when they have fresh donuts in your area.

Food producers have us and our triggers figured out to get us to buy their products. Food habits are primal, and not easy to change once adopted. We no longer learn what to eat from watching our mother's prepare food, but from watching commercials. We're bombarded with food advertising. Food manufacturers perfectly tweak their products to light up the food addiction centers in the brain.

For example, in food commercials, a food artist prepares perfect burgers. The commercial is shot from the perspective of the viewer, as if you were biting into the grilled-to-perfection burger, making it even more irresistible. Nothing like a juicy, cheesy, bacon-laden burger staring you in the face to trigger a quick trip to the nearest burger joint.

> *It's amazing how pervasive food is. Every second commercial is for food. Every second TV episode takes place around a meal. In the city, you can't go ten feet without seeing or smelling a restaurant. There are 20-foot-high hamburgers up on billboards. I am acutely aware of food, and its omnipresence is astounding.*
>
> —ADAM SCOTT, VIDEO BLOGGER, THE MONKEY CHOW DIARIES

## HOW DO YOU RESIST CRAVINGS?

Cravings are a neurological mechanism where hormones and other chemicals percolate from the gut, moving up the vagus nerve into the brain. The brain then cranks up the release of dopamine, a compound related to reward-motivation behavior, and drives up the intensity of the desire and reward. The resulting urge to eat whatever particular food has spurred the craving is linked to a brain process controlled by leptin. Leptin is a hormone released after a meal that creates the sense of satisfaction and fullness. Your belly may be bulging with turkey and stuffing, but when the pecan pie is placed on the table, the leptin mumbles, "No," but the dopamine causes the reward-motivation center of your brain to screams, "Go for it!"

"Researchers have discovered a real and entirely unexpected bonus to resisting the cravings-driven urge to consume junk," says John Apolzan, PhD, a nutrition scientist at Louisiana State University: if you can kick the objects of your cravings out of your diet, even for just a few weeks, the cravings start to fade. "Earlier research suggested cravings should skyrocket when you resist them," says Apolzan. "But now it's clear that's just not true." The reason they diminish is that cravings are the product of habit—the more often you give into your cravings, the stronger and more fixed they become. "Changing your habits seems to reverse the process," says Apolzan.

> *An ounce of prevention is worth a pound of cure.*
> —BENJAMIN FRANKLIN

## FOOD PRODUCTS ARE NOT REAL FOOD

Food advertising is pervasive, and for a good reason: profits. Coca-Cola spends approximately $9.25 per person living in the United States because we spend roughly $452 per person annually on their products.

Processed food is a business, and businesses need you to spend your money. We don't see commercials for broccoli. The ripest, juiciest peach is not as addictive as a sugar-laden bowl of breakfast cereal. The question is, are food manufacturers giving people what they want, or are they engineering food to tap into our primal instincts and cravings?

Processed food can mean many things. Frozen organic spinach in a bag is a form of processed food. Minimally processed food like organic frozen fruits and vegetables are convenient and good to keep on hand. It's the food items that are heavily processed, going through a series of mechanical and chemical engineering, that are concerning.

Highly processed foods usually contain cheap fats such as vegetable oils that are generally hard to digest, along with salt, sugars, and other heavily refined carbohydrates, that have been stripped of their bran, fiber, and nutrients.

There's an additional concern with carbs, like corn, wheat, and soybeans. They've been sprayed with chemical weed killers, and the effect of those chemicals on the body may be damaging. For example, white bread is made of heavily refined flour stripped of nutrients and fiber, and the wheat growth was probably managed with weed-killing chemicals.

Even in 430 BC, Hippocrates described the laxative effects of course wheat compared with refined wheat.[38]

Eating food is usually something we do several times a day. The most fundamental reason to eat is to nourish your body. Good health and nourishment are as much about what you don't eat as what you do eat. We tend to concern ourselves with calories first, but it's a matter of nutritional content too. Draw a line between this important distinction, now and forever.

When it comes to processed foods that are calorie-rich and nutritionally void, there are three food traits to ditch from your diet:

## 1. Highly Refined Grains

Refining grains strips out both the bran and the germ to give the product a finer texture and, most importantly to food manufacturers, a longer shelf life. The refining also removes many nutrients. Examples of these nutritionally void, highly processed grains are white bread, some kinds of pasta, many cereals, white rice, and any grain that has been enriched. Because of the refinement, these products quickly turn into glucose, hit your body's processing system like a freight train, and spike blood glucose levels. The body's processing system is not designed to handle these spikes long term.

## 2. Added Sugar

As we discussed, so many manufactured food products contain

boatloads of added sugar. This is apparent in some products, like candy, cakes, and cookies. Still, there are many you may not necessarily know have added sugars, like peanut butter, spaghetti sauce, ketchup, salad dressing, and protein bars. Remember, there are at least fifty-six different names for sugars, most commonly cane sugar and high-fructose corn syrup. All sugars have little to no nutritional value. Even natural sugars offer such small amounts of vitamins and minerals in comparison to other foods that you could easily do without them. It's best to limit all sugar intake and choose natural sugars or whole-foods like fruits that contain natural sugars to satisfy your sweet tooth.

## 3. Vegetable Oils

If the oil comes from something that is not oily, like canola, soybean, corn, safflower, margarine, sunflower, and hydrogenated fats, then ditch it. These oils are damaged during the extensive caustic refining process, which causes the oils to oxidize and create those harmful free radicals. New York Times best-selling author and highly regarded wellness expert, Ben Greenfield, states that these oils are worse than sugar.

In prehistoric times, our genetic predisposition for calorie-rich foods may have helped us pack on extra calories to survive the possibility of famines during those hunter-gatherer years. At times, early man faced episodes of famine and food scarcities. Today, in a country like the United States, it's hard to imagine food scarcity, but our genetics have not evolved enough, and we still have the same food cravings.

The manufacturers of food products have our predisposition for the calorie-rich foods full of fat and sugar in their crosshairs. As mere mortals, we'll have a hard time trying to outsmart our ancestral genetics or the multibillion-dollar food industry. In modern life, we're surrounded by fast-food restaurants, advertisements of cheap calories, all-you-can-eat buffets, and food beckoning us twenty-four hours a day. Even going grocery shopping, we're faced with temptation on every aisle.

Our hectic lifestyle plays into the need for convenient food, and the food industries hope they can engineer the tastes to keep you coming back for more. As a potato chip commercial stated, "You can't eat just one."

> *Fast food is popular because it's convenient. It's cheap, and it tastes good. But the real cost of eating fast food never appears on the menu.*
> —ERIC SCHLOSSER, AUTHOR, FAST FOOD NATION

## FOOD ROOTS: EAT LIKE YOUR GREAT-GRANDMA

My cousins lived on a rural farm and my father was raised on a farm in southern Missouri. Although I grew up in the city, we visited my cousins' farm often. My father's food-roots philosophy was, grow it, hunt it, catch it, clean it, cook it, and eat it.

**Food roots: everything that happens to your food before you eat it.**

If you wanted chicken for dinner, you went to the chicken coop. If you wanted corn, you sneaked into your neighbor's cornfield with a bucket. The ice cream was cranked by hand and the cream came from a local farmer's cow. Thanksgiving, you went hunting for a turkey. You baked bread, grew beans, canned tomatoes, and made jams. You knew where your food came from, how your food was made, and who made your food.

We're so far removed from the concept of a chicken coop in the backyard. Today, our chicken comes wrapped in plastic on a bed of Styrofoam. Logos on the packaging feature happy cartoon chickens with red barns to make us feel like we have some connection with rural Americana. But in actuality, we have no connection with the animal that was killed for our consumption.

Food roots put you in contact with your food sources. Where was the food grown? How was it grown? How was it processed? What was sprayed on it? How was it packaged and shipped? What chemicals were added? So many questions need answers and your awareness.

In a typical chain-restaurant hamburger, you might also find sodium nitrates (a coloring agent), sodium benzoate, (a preservative), sulfites, (also a preservative), carbon monoxide, (pigmentation aid), bacteria from fecal matter (shit happens), pesticides, (chemicals sprayed on crops the cow eats), and other substances.[39] Yet, we blindly put chemicals in our body that if we truly understand the effects, we probably would make very different choices. It's awareness of your food's roots that can help you make a difference in what you feed your body.

For the first time in history, life expectancy has shifted to a downward trend. Our children are not expected to live as long as us. More than a third of Americans are living with diabetes or prediabetes and face the severe complications that can arise from this disease.

Food-related diseases include heart disease, stroke, diabetes, and cancers. These and other diseases are the leading causes of death in the United States and are largely preventable through diet and other supporting factors like exercise and sleep.

Diets are nothing new. For decades, we've been on the hunt for easy weight-loss strategies that will shed the unwanted, unhealthy pounds, but they all focus on calorie restriction instead of nutrient inclusion. Real foods have vitamins, minerals, phytonutrients, and naturally occurring fats, sugars, and proteins the body craves and needs for sustained optimum health. These nutrient-dense foods are the winners when choosing a diet to shed pounds. Remember the diversity of the gut microbiome depended on a diverse variety of foods and was key to weight management.

William Banting first popularized the concept of dieting in 1863 with a pamphlet published on his diet strategy called *Letter on Corpulence, Addressed to the Public.* It was the first published guide on dieting for weight loss and set out the weight-loss plan Banting used to address his own obesity.

Banting was an eminent funeral director in London. Overseeing the funerals of King George III and King George IV, as well as other royals, put him in the spotlight of the London elite. So did his portly, obese appearance. After he shed the pounds, his slim presence was noted, and his weight-loss strategy became popular with the general public. Like most diets, Banting's method was to restrict carbohydrates of starches and sugars.

Since Banting, well over a century ago, many are still in search of an easy way to lose weight. Although genetics, your gut microbiome and your metabolism are all factors that may impair weight loss, simply put, if you consume more food than your body can use, you will gain weight. To lose that weight, there almost always needs to be a deficit of calories. The question is, Does what you eat matter more than how much you eat?

Both are right, but it's not that simple.

There's an array of diet strategies out there. Some profess everything from eating like our prehistoric ancestors to eliminating somethings specific—no carbs, no fat, no wheat, no sugar, no nightshade vegetables, no this, no that, until you're left with a bowl of ice for dinner. Instead of focusing on the negative, I suggest starting with the positive. Here's why.

The word *diet* evokes restrictions. The definition of a diet is a special course of food to which one restricts oneself, either to lose weight or for medical reasons. Humans don't like limitations. We rebel. We might be successful at following a diet at first, but statistics show diets are rarely successful long term. Sadly, roughly 90 percent of people who lose weight eventually gain it all back—and sometimes, gained even more.

What works long term is a commitment to an overall healthy lifestyle. Ask yourself, Does 90 percent of what you eat serve your future self or not? Lifestyle is defined as the way in which a person lives. It's a commitment to a way of life and a way of eating—but it has to be simple.

## THREE SIMPLE RULES FOR YOUR FOOD LIFESTYLE

Michael Pollan, in the documentary titled *In Defense of Food,* boils healthy eating down to three simple rules:

1. Eat real food.
2. Not too much.
3. Mostly plants.

These simple rules align with humans being omnivores, meaning we can digest both plant and animal products. The digestive tracts of carnivores are shorter than ours, and their stomachs have a higher acid content to break down the animal products rapidly. The short digestive tracts absorb the nutrients, then swiftly moves the digested matter along for elimination, avoiding the possibility of purification in the intestines. Herbivores digestive tracts are much longer to give time to break down the cell walls of plant material. Humans are in between, but do better with a plant-rich diet.

People can choose to be vegan for a variety of reasons, but the most important consideration for our diet is that our food be real, not packaged, manipulated food products dreamt up by food manufacturers. Broccoli is broccoli. Sautéed with salt and pepper, maybe a little lemon juice—it's delicious. Why drink processed apple juice when you can eat an apple? A medium-sized apple is about the same 100 calories as an eight-ounce cup of apple juice. Which would give you more satiation and fill you up? Apple juice floods your system with liquid sugar, whereas an apple is loaded with plant material, fibers, phytonutrients and gives your stomach something to work on. We need to change our eating habits and go for the whole food, not its parts.

*You must unlearn what you have learned.*
—YODA, MOST POWERFUL MEMBER OF THE JEDI ORDER, STAR WARS

# VEGAN: GOING ALL IN

I can't complete a chapter on food without discussing a vegan lifestyle and the reasoning why you might consider it.

All protein originates from plant material. Take a look at a cow's diet: it's plant based. All the protein you get from eating a steak came from the plant source the cow ate. The same is true with all the meats humans eat— whether chickens, pigs, or lamb. These animals are just the middleman for protein sources.

In other words, you don't need to get your protein from animal sources to get adequate protein in your diet. Most meat eaters get about half their protein from consuming plants anyway. One cup of lentils or a peanut butter sandwich has about the same amount of protein as three ounces of beef or three eggs.

The reason we need protein is protein is made up of strings of amino acids—the building blocks of life—and nine are essential amino acids that our bodies can't make and need to get from our food sources. All plants contain the nine essential amino acids in varying proportions. As long as you consume the proper amount of these amino acids, the source is irrelevant.

Another fallacy is you need high amounts of animal proteins to build stronger bodies and develop powerful muscle, like in the case of an elite athlete. This, too, is wrong. Muscles run on glycogen, which comes from carbohydrates. Carbohydrates are broken down by the body into a type of sugar called glucose. Glycogen is a branched polymer form of glucose stored in the muscles and liver. Glycogen is the fuel for the muscles, especially during rigorous exercise.

Many elite athletes are vegans and promote the vegan diet as the primary tool that catapulted their training to win record-breaking competitions. Several vegans have won places on the podium at the Olympic Games: figure skater Meagan Duhamel won silver, bobsledder Alexey Voevoda won two gold, cyclist Dotsie Bausch won silver, Carl Lewis has won ten Olympic medals over his career—the list goes on. Scott Jurek, ultra-marathoner ran the Appalachian trail—all 2,189 miles of it—in the record time of forty-six days, averaging over fifty miles per day. Patrik Babumian, the strongest man in the world, stopped eating meat in 2005 and went from 105 kilos to 130 kilos and set four world records. When he stopped eating meat, he got bigger and stronger. To set the world record, he carried 1,244 pounds for thirty-three feet.[40]

Ephesus, Turkey, the most preserved city of the ancient Romans, dates back to the second and third century BC. Recent archeological digs uncovered the graves of sixty-eight gladiators. To get an idea of their diet, the bones were examined for mineral content. High levels of strontium were found, which indicates a vegetarian diet; low amounts would mean a carnivore's diet. Further study of their bones found they endured high standards of training that built strong bones and muscles but ate a diet of high-quality grains and beans.[41]

The biological functions that made gladiators and all these champion athletes strong also affect our health, specifically in terms of chronic inflammation, oxidative damage, and endothelial function. An animal-based diet may have an adverse effect on the gut microbiome, showing an overgrowth of bacterial species that promote inflammation. When animal proteins are ingested, our gut bacteria form inflammatory compounds that adversely affect the lining of our blood vessels, creating inflammation and restricting blood flow. Also, the inflammatory compounds tend to rev up our cells to multiply faster, which can lead to a higher risk of cancers.[42]

A whole-food, plant-based diet can decrease blood pressure, cholesterol, and inflammation markers and therefore is a proven diet to prevent, treat, and possible reverse heart disease. Plant-based diets optimize new growth of blood vessels in damaged tissues, repairing muscles and tendons.[43]

Furthermore, antioxidants, substances that may protect your cells against the effects of free radical damage, are found almost entirely in plants. Plus, plant-based foods can reduce inflammation by 30 percent over three weeks.

Eating plant based not only helps the body, it also helps the planet. At a considerable cost to biodiversity, three-quarters of all agricultural land is used for livestock production. Meat, dairy, egg, and fish farming use 83 percent of the world's resources, including 27 percent of all freshwater, for only 18 percent of the world's calories.

| HOW MUCH WATER NEEDED TO PRODUCE OUR FOOD? | |
| --- | --- |
| **PER POUND** | **GALLONS OF WATER** |
| Animal Agriculture | |
| **1 Pound of Beef** | **13,000 Gallons** |
| **1 Pound of Pork** | **3,000 Gallons** |
| **1 Pound of Chicken** | **2,340 Gallons** |
| | |
| Dairy | |
| **1 Pound of Cheese** | **3,000 Gallons** |
| **1 Gallon of Milk** | **3,780 Gallons** |
| | |
| Grains | |
| **1 Pound of Rice** | **2,200 Gallons** |
| **1 Pound of Corn or Wheat** | **750 Gallons** |

Animals eat the grains and water, plus they have land needs. The pre-cow process of raising the grains involves spraying them with herbicides, which run off into our water supplies, and the post-cow problems include the cow's waste of leaching into the water supply. Animal agriculture in the United States produced fifty times more waste of urine and feces per year than the waste of the entire human population. And, raising cattle for beef and dairy products contributes to climate change. Cows produce methane gas and nitrous oxide as byproducts from digestion and manure. Worldwide, all livestock accounts for 14.5 percent of greenhouse gas emissions.[44]

The 2019, Healy Around the World Barcelona conference decided their gala dinner would be all vegan, plant-based food. During the dinner an announcement was made that they used a vegan online calculator to calculate how the dinner impacted consumption of water and animals. What would you guess?

The answer: two million liters of water and 545 animals were saved.

The evidence is overwhelming: the more plants you eat, the healthier you will be, and so will the environment.

Many illnesses today are food related, but the food industry doesn't want you to focus on that. The food manufacturers are in the business of manufacturing desire. They want you to believe you will be happier and healthier by consuming their products. Slogans like "meat does a body good" try to persuade you to buy into the dream that if you eat their product, your life will be better.

Arby's claims, "It's good mood food" and "We have the meats."
McDonald's, "You deserve a break today."
Wendy's, "Where's the beef?"
And the beef industry, "Beef—it's what's for dinner."
And the dairy industry, "Milk does a body good," and "Got milk?"

A good slogan or jingle is designed to stay with you—even for decades. Slogans and jingles are simple, memorable, and most importantly, recognizable when you're faced with making choices. They become your go-to friend. Marketing by food manufacturers are no different. Remember, food is a business, and the manufacturers want you to buy their product. You only need to walk the aisles of the grocery store, pick up a product, and imagine what went into making it. Even something as simple as steak has a backstory that's not apparent as you stand there deciding on strip steak or rib eye.

## THE 70 PERCENT VEGAN APPROACH

There are so many reasons to go vegan. A whole-food, plant-based diet has been shown to be a key factor in optimal health. If you're having a hard time going cold turkey on animal products, consider an approach that I call the 70 percent vegan.

Look at your plate of food. Is 70 percent plant based? Eating a spinach salad with vegetables is a wise choice, but some people look at a plate of spinach and retreat. What if your salad had two of pieces of crumbled bacon sprinkled on it? Would that be enticing enough to want to eat it? Then do that for now. After a while, maybe you'll ditch the bacon. In the meantime, you will be eating more plant foods.

My go-to breakfast drink contains filtered water, ten ounces of spinach, a little lemon juice, and a small piece of fruit like an apple or a pear. I put it through a high-speed blender until it's a green smoothie. The fruit makes the spinach taste unnoticeable. Now I have the nutritional advantage of eating a spinach salad and the hydration of all that fluid. It's a great way to start your 70 percent vegan day.

We eat every day and cooking is the most useful life skill you could learn. You'll use it your entire life. Spend the time to watch cooking shows, search easy recipes online, and develop a repertoire of break-fast, lunch, and dinner recipes. Being able to cook and prepare healthy meals gives you freedom of choice and can save you money. You truly can have it your way.

## CHAPTER SUMMARY

☑ Take a probiotic with a diverse amount of microorganism to balance your gut microbiome.

☑ Ditch processed foods manufactured with refined grains, added sugar and heavily processed oils.

☑ Learn to cook ten healthy, tasty recipes. Try different options for breakfast, lunch and dinner. Use as many fruits and vegetables as possible.

☑ Follow the three simple rules: Eat real food. Not too much. Mostly plants.

☑ Does what you eat serve your healthy lifestyle? Does it serve your future self?

☑ Make sure at least 70 percent of your food comes from fruits, vegetables, nuts, seeds, and legumes, with the remaining 30 percent or less coming from animal products.

☑ Know your food roots. Know where your food comes from and what's happened to it before you eat it. Is it organic or sprayed with harmful chemicals?

## CHAPTER SEVEN

# Sleep, Perchance to Dream

*And God blessed the seventh day, and sanctified*
*it: because that in it he had rested from all*
*his work which God created and made.*
—THE KING JAMES BIBLE

In ancient societies, dreams foretold futures, set social standards, and created myths and Gods. Early nineteenth-century psychoanalysts like Sigmund Freud claimed dreams reflected our repressed selves. It's tough to know what dreams are about, as it's challenging to study the dream process. You have to wake the person up to ask them questions, thus disturbing the very thing you are attempting to study.

We do know if we sleep well, we have an improved waking experience. We also know that during sleep, some crazy, wild stuff goes on in our head that we call dreaming. Sleep must be incredibly important as we spend almost a third of our lives in this altered state of consciousness.

**We are such stuff as dreams are made on.**
—WILLIAM SHAKESPEARE

Sleep is one of the body's most basic needs, like breathing, food, and water—you would die without it.

When sleep deprived for a day, the body undergoes subtle changes. The levels of the hormone cortisol and thyroid-stimulating hormone (TSH) increase, leading to a rise in blood pressure. A few days later, glucose stops metabolizing properly, leading to carbohydrate cravings. This may also be one of the contributing factors to obesity in people who are sleep deprived. The body temperature drops, and the immune system becomes suppressed. There's nothing life-threatening within the first few days, and any negative effects are reversible with extended catch-up sleep. But what would happen if we continued without sleep?

In the 1980s, a series of sleep deprivation studies were conducted on rats. After thirty-two days, all the rats were dead. Several possible causes were put forward: the rat's body temperature dropped so dramatically they all died from hypothermia. Or the normal gut bacteria spread throughout the bodies, and the immune systems were too depressed to fight the reaction. The rats also showed evidence of brain damage, or the extreme levels of stress, with all the other related factors, could have been the demise of the rats.

Our knowledge of sleep deprivation in humans is limited because not only would prolonged sleep deprivation for scientific study be cruel, who would volunteer for a potentially deadly study? There have been studies limited to three days of sleep deprivation that show psychological effects such as hallucinations and paranoia. The period is too short to experience severe physical symptoms, but I think it is safe to assume we probably wouldn't do much better than the rats if sleep deprived for weeks or months.[45]

During sleep deprivation, brain cells have difficulty communicating, cognitive performance worsens, and fatigue sets in. While sleep requirements vary from person to person, most adults need seven to nine hours of sleep a night. This has to do with one's circadian rhythm.

Your circadian rhythm is an internal clock running in the background of your brain that regulates intervals of sleepiness and alertness during a twenty-four-hour day. Since it's a rhythm, it's best to have regular sleep and waking habits. It's a good idea to go to sleep and wake at the same time every day, including weekends.

Our need for sleep adjusts with age. Babies and children need more sleep than older adults. For this chapter on sleep, we'll focus on the part of your circadian rhythm that happens during the seven to nine hours of sleep most of us should be getting each night.

> *Go to bed. You'll feel better tomorrow. is the human version of, "Did you try turning it off and on again?"*
> —ANONYMOUS

Sleep is a naturally recurring state required for the body and the mind to rejuvenate. Our body goes into a form of hibernation where our senses are inhibited, nearly all voluntary muscle movement ceases, and our interactions with our surroundings are reduced. Our consciousness goes into an altered state. We spend our night cycling through two states of sleep: non-rapid eye movement (NREM) and rapid eye movement (REM) sleep.

The NREM sleep, is broken down into three stages. These stages aid the transition between the body becoming inactive, and the brain becoming active.

In the first stage, you still have a sense of awareness, can still hear things, and don't feel like you're asleep. This stage is usually short lived. This is the 20 minutes or so when you first go to bed.

By the second stage, also called light sleep, you're asleep but could easily be awakened. Sometimes you feel a sensation of falling that jolts you back awake. This stage of sleep takes up more than half the night as we cycle back and forth through this second stage of NREM and REM. Our body starts the repair process of regulating metabolism and sorting memories and emotions.

By the third stage of NREM, also called the deep sleep stage, you're in a deep sleep, but not dreaming yet. The body has relaxed. This stage of deep sleep accounts for approximately 18 to 20 percent of the sleep. Deep sleep is associated with cellular repair and strengthening your immune system. The body is most active in its repair process during this stage.

And finally, we've passed through the three stages of NREM into the REM state. If deep NREM sleep is about the body, REM is about the brain. The brain becomes the most active during REM sleep, so active that chemicals are released through the body to relax and slightly paralyze the muscles. The paralysis puts your body offline so you don't act out your dreams.

The body is most active during the three stages of NREM. For the brain, it's the opposite. The brain fires up when you enter REM sleep. During REM sleep, the brain goes from consciousness to an altered consciousness. The brainwaves have slowed, and it's much harder to wake up.

Full REM is the last and deepest stage of sleep. Your eyes dart back and forth behind your eyelids—thus, the name rapid eye movement sleep. It's the REM stage where your brain fires up and is as active as when you're completely awake. Unlike NREM with three stages, REM has only one stage.

During the night, the brain cycles in and out of the REM sleep, with the first cycle occurring approximately ninety minutes after sleep has started. This is when dreams happen. According to the National Sleep Foundation, REM sleep makes up about 25 percent of your sleeping time. You cycle in and out of the REM sleep about every ninety minutes, but as the night goes on, the REM sleep become deeper, longer, and more active.

Since REM sleep doesn't even start until you've slept for about ninety minutes, the seven to nine hours of recommended sleep will get you three to five cycles through the REM sleep. Burning the candle at both ends—going to bed late and getting up early—cuts into your ability to get into the REM sleep, the most restorative stage of sleep, and lessens the depth and time you spend in REM.

You can think of REM sleep and NREM deep sleep as the two most restorative parts of sleep. The rest is light sleep, which takes up about 50 percent of the night. The current thinking is whether you get more or less light sleep isn't really going to matter or affect how you feel the next day but in the future research may uncover more about the function of light sleep.[46]

The two main causes of less sleep are age—people tend to get less of restorative sleep as they get older—and anything that interferes with your sleep, like pain, illness, medication, sleep apnea, other sleep disorders, or working night shifts, which disrupts the natural cycle of sleep.

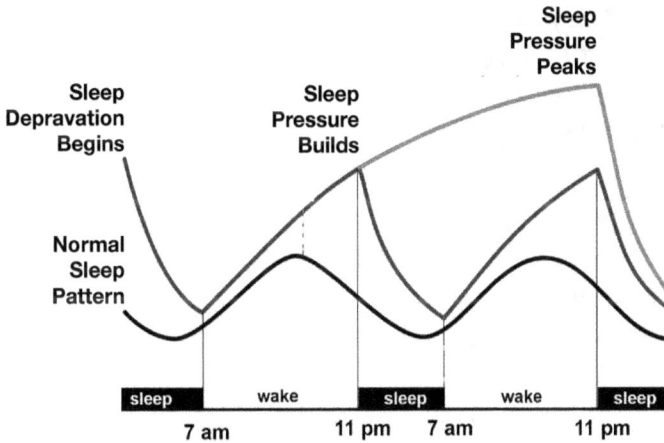

## CIRCADIAN RHYTHM
### NORMAL SLEEP AND OF SLEEP DEPRAVATION

The body needs sleep to rejuvenate, grow muscle and repair tissues. Sleep affects our ability to synthesize hormones. Sleep also plays a vital role in the brain's ability to sort and store information and consolidate memories. People who get adequate sleep tend to retain information and perform better on cognitive and memory tasks. During sleep, the body and brain go into the repair shop, and wash away toxins and waste products. Tissues repair themselves, and energy stores are replenished.

*A good laugh and a long sleep are the
two best cures for anything.*
−IRISH PROVERB

If you want to get more REM sleep, follow these steps:

1. Avoid these sleep-wreakers: stimulants such as caffeine and nicotine six hours before sleep; alcohol, which can also interfere with the REM stage: and heavy meals before bed, which affects sleep and digestion.
2. Stick to a regular sleep schedule. Go to bed and wake at the same time every day. To get the full benefits of REM sleep, go to bed early enough to let the body have the time to wake on its own without an alarm.
3. Exercise.
4. Make your bedroom a sleep sanctuary—a cool, dark room with no TV, computers, or cell phones.

## DRUNK SLEEPING

Although not illegal, driving while sleep deprived can be worse than driving drunk. A study from AAA shows driving on less than five hours of sleep is the same as driving drunk. Drowsy driving is estimated to be a factor in 20 percent of fatal crashes.[47]

Drivers who are fatigued or sleep deprived experience what is known as microsleep. Microsleep is extremely brief periods of falling asleep—from a half second to possible ten seconds—and these tiny gaps in awareness makes micro sleep dangerous. When you're driving a vehicle the size of an elephant, even a split-second can be disastrous.

A car going 55 mph travels about eighty feet every second. It doesn't take more than a half second of shut-eye for the situation to become deadly, especially when you add the perception and reaction time for the brain to catch up once you open your eyes again. Microsleep and fatigue is the number one problem for sleep-deprived drivers. Coffee or other simulants will not solve the problem. The only remedy is sleep.

**When the going gets tough, the tough go take a nap.**
−TOM HODGKINSON, BRITISH WRITER

Sleepless nights hurt. There's a cost in lost productivity. Work-related injuries are higher, and those who consistently go without sleep are more likely to have health-related problems. If our zombie mode is doing so much damage, then what happens when we are well rested?

A new study suggests sleep makes a monumental difference. Two groups of researchers from universities in Belgium surveyed 621 students regarding their sleep habits during exams. The grades of students who slept seven hours a night were 10 percent higher than those of the students who went into the exams sleep deprived.

"New knowledge is integrated into our existing knowledge base while we sleep," said researcher Dr.Stijin Baert.

Students who get adequate sleep, have better-quality sleep, and keep the consistent habit patterns of their sleep tend to do better on tests. It takes all three—duration, quality, and consistency. According to the study results, the quality of sleep seemed linked to bedtime. A bedtime between 10:00 p.m. and 1:00 a.m. but no later seemed to be the sweet spot for inducing better-quality sleep.

## DREAM MACHINE

Keith Richards woke one morning to find the cassette player by his bed had a recording on it. Apparently, he had awakened in the middle of the night and recorded the legendary riff and the words to "(I Can't

Get No) Satisfaction." Similar stories emerged from Beatles members Paul McCartney and John Lennon, plus other rock gods.

**The nicest thing for me is sleep. Then at least I can dream.**
−MARILYN MONROE

Creative people may remember more of their dreams, and because they're creative they may use what happens at night as inspiration for their day. Most people dream several times a night, but the average person remembers about half their dreams, and others have no dream recall at all. One study showed that people who were more prone to absorption, imaginativeness, daydreaming, and fantasizing were most likely to remember their dreams.

"There is a fundamental continuity between how people experience the world during the day and at night," said University of Iowa psychology professor David Watson. "People who are prone to daydreaming and fantasy have less of a barrier between states of sleep and wakefulness and seem to pass between them more easily."[48]

Lucid dreaming is a dream during which the dreamer is aware they are dreaming. Many lucid dreamers can even control or change the narrative of their dreams to create a pleasant dream instead of succumbing to a nightmare. If nightmares or fears come up, lucid dreamers know they're not in the real world and safely explore their fears without feeling threat-ened. And for some, lucid dreams are an outpouring of the adventurous spirit, taking on superpowers they would not be able to do or traveling to places they wouldn't be able to go to in real life.

**Sleep is the best meditation.**
−DALAI LAMA, BUDDHIST SPIRITUAL LEADER

There's a phenomenon that happens in our sleep called sleep paralysis. It's more common at the beginning of the night when we're falling asleep and at the end when we are waking for the day. During this paralyzed state, we may feel the presence of an individual, pressure on the body holding us down, or feelings of out-of-body floating where your spirit has left your body. It may feel ominous not to be able to move, but it will pass within a few minutes. This is where our rational mind can rest assured the little green men are not out to get us, and it's just a momentary lapse caused by sleep paralysis.

For most of us, sleep is often cut short to accommodate our busy lives, but this isn't healthy in the long run. A few days of sleep deprivation to get a project launched or take care of an ill child is understandable. But sleep needs to be a priority for your overall health and well-being. It's not optional, even for minimum health, and it's mandatory for optimal health. Getting more restorative sleep is totally doable.

*Learn from yesterday, live for today,*
*look to tomorrow, rest this afternoon.*
—CHARLES M. SCHULZ, CREATOR, PEANUTS COMIC

## THE WITCHING HOUR

For many of us, the hour around bedtime is the most challenging time of day or night. It's time we need to wind down and get ready for bed. The time to shut off the endless list of stuff to do and just let go.

For example, many people turn the TV on as soon as they walk in the door of their home, having it always on in the background. The average person in the US watches about five hours of television per day, which adds up to thirty-five hours each week.[49] This is nearly the number of hours that would have been spent on a full-time job. Having the TV always on is not only a bad idea for the house, but it's also a disastrous idea for the bedroom and sleep. The TV is people talking which is a constant distraction. The brain has to pay attention to what is being said. Even if you're not actually paying attention but listening passively, the sound of people talking is work for the brain. There's no peace. The brain needs to wind down and rest, especially before bed.

> **The lion and the calf shall lie down together,**
> **but the calf won't get much sleep.**
> —WOODY ALLEN

Sixty-four percent of households have a TV in the bedroom. The claims are that the white noise of the television helps them sleep. Television is entertaining and enjoyable at the end of the day—you can catch up on the news or the latest TV show. That sounds fine, but research has proven much differently.

*Binge-watching* is a relatively new term that arose because of the wide array of entertainment sources now available—Netflix, Amazon and cable. Time is our most limited resource and watching TV shows can be very time consuming, making a TV in the bedroom possibly one of the worst decisions you can make. Watching TV can rob you of sleep, your physical and emotional health, and the health of your relationship with your partner or spouse.

Television in the bedroom impairs beneficial sleep. Someone is always talking or imparting information, a story is requiring our attention, or advertisements are selling us products. We're more likely to purchase things when we are tired or bored. Television is not reality, and TV shows are not accurate depictions of the world. We can become disillusioned about the expectations of our life when our lives don't measure up to what we see on the TV.

Social media is another source of false perceptions and unhealthy distractions that can affect sleep. FOMO—"fear of missing out."—is a side effect of the boom in social media. If you somehow missed the meaning of this acronym, it describes that feeling of anxiety we may experience when we see other people having fun together or doing something special without us. It can be a brief, passing pang of envy, or instill real self-doubts and feelings of inadequacy. We might feel we've missed an opportunity. Online networks make it instantly possible to compare ourselves and our lives to others. Is this how you want to end your day? Are these the thoughts you want haunting your dreams? Probably not. Ban social media in the hours before bed.

Why is it bad for you and your marriage or partnership?

When it comes to bedtime and mornings, what you think last and first matters. It's when the brain is most open to suggestability—the inclination to accept and act on the suggestions of others, whether its beneficial or not. An action movie or a murder mystery before bed has your brain marinating in sleep-disruptive content. Instead, before bed try contemplating your day's activities, writing in a journal, laying out your clothes or doing other things to prep for the day ahead.

*Take rest: a field that has rested gives bountiful crop.*
—OVID, 43 BC, ANCIENT ROMAN POET

Upon waking, set the stage for your day and your thoughts yourself rather than allowing some television show, countless emails, or news program to paint your thoughts for you. Healthier, authentic thoughts can flourish when you have the distraction-free space to let them. Use the extra time to stretch for ten minutes, make a healthy breakfast, or meditate. It's time: use it for yourself instead of allowing the useless chatter of TV, social media or emails to guide your thoughts and actions.

For your marriage or snuggling with that special someone, the waning and waking hours affords couples time for togetherness, evoke more intimacy with conversation, and provide more sexual opportunities— without the distraction of the latest sports update. Statistics show couples who have a television in the bedroom have sex half as often as those who don't. That should be reason enough to ditch the TV. What could be better between couples than providing the opportunity for cuddling, conversations, light humor, sex, and developing the intimate bond of love? The bedroom is the perfect place for intimacy to grow.

*You know you're in love when you can't fall asleep*
*because reality is finally better than your dreams.*
—DR. SEUSS

Repeat after me.

No TV in the bedroom, no cell phone, no computer. Nada.

The bedroom needs to be an anxiety-free space. Free of distractions, and that means no TV, computer, or phone. I know people use their phone for an alarm, but they still make clocks for that. Or turn the phone on silent mode—so no buzzing, clicking, or beeping—and place it face down on the surface, far enough away so you would have to get out of bed to pick it up.

Above all else, the bedroom needs to be a sanctuary. Here are some doable steps to creating your sanctuary:

## 1. Hello Darkness, My Old Friend
Bring the room to its nearest level of darkness by closing the drapes and turning off all light sources, even the soft lights and LED lights from electronics. If you're unable to make it completely dark, consider using a sleep mask. The darkness promotes your body's ability to produce melatonin, a hormone that promotes restful sleep.

## 2. Keep Cool, Baby
During the night, the body's temperature drops. Set the thermostat or open a window for the bedroom temperature to be between 60 and 68 degrees, which is the ideal temperature for sleep.

### 3. Silence is Golden

Extraneous noise can jar you awake or prevent you from falling asleep. Noise interruptions through the night affect your quality of sleep and your ability to move from lighter sleep into deep restorative sleep. If you can't control the sounds around you, a white noise machine or earplugs can help block out noise.

### 4. Comfort is King

The quality of your mattress, pillow, blankets, and even your pajamas—or going commando, without pajamas—matters. Are your PJs 100 percent breathable cotton or polyester? Do your sheets feel comforting as you slide into bed? Do your mattress and pillow support your body's needs? Most quality mattresses last only about ten years before they start to lose their support. Is your pillow down, hard foam, or sponge? All these things matter to your comfort.

### 5. Decluttered Means Destressed

Sometimes the space around our bed becomes a dump zone for projects, clothes, laundry, storage, exercise equipment, and other stuff. We are visual beings, and what we see is essential to the quality of our thoughts. A stress-free, decluttered bedroom sets the mind to sanctuary mode, ready to enjoy the night's sleep ahead.

## SNORE NO MORE

Snoring happens when you can't move air freely through your mouth or your nose down into your lungs. The mouth and the nose are the only two ways we can get air into our lungs, so clear passageways are essential. When we sleep, tissues around the back of the throat, tongue, and nasal area become relaxed and can flop around as the air moves in and out, causing the vibrational snoring. There are several contributors to snoring, including excess weight around the mouth or throat, the way you're built, nasal or sinus problems, alcohol, smoking or medications, and your sleep posture.

Snoring could be a sign of a more serious sleep disorder, such as sleep apnea, but only a qualified sleep therapist or doctor can make that determination. If your snoring comes with sleep apnea, which involves the cessation of breath for more than ten seconds, you may want to seek medical advice.

**Laugh and the world laughs with you.**
**Snore, and you sleep alone.**
—ANTHONY BURGESS, ENGLISH WRITER

There are a few home remedies to try to eliminate or reduce snoring. One, change your sleep posture. Elevating your head four to six inches may make breathing easier. Sleeping on your side and not your back also may help clear the airways. There are anti-snoring mouth appliances—mouth guards—that manipulate the upper and lower jaw, keeping the tongue or throat tissues out of the air passageway. You can keep your sinus passages clear with a saline solution nasal rinse before bed or a decongestant if needed.

## SOOTHE YOUR SNORING BEAST

As I said earlier, my personal favorite for stopping my own snoring is taping my mouth shut. Remember—not my entire mouth but a half-inch piece of paper tape that goes vertically down the center of my mouth from just below my nose to my chin. This keeps my mouth gently closed while still allowing me to cough out both sides my mouth if needed, and the tape is easily removed. In addition, I wear earplugs and a cloth bandana over my eyes. It may look like a hostage crisis in my bedroom—It's definitely not my sexiest look—but the technique of an eye wrap, earplugs, and taping my mouth partially shut has provided me deep, restful, and restorative sleep.

By partially taping the mouth shut, you're forced to breathe through the nasal passageway. As I mentioned in the chapter on breathing, breath through the sinus adds nitric oxide to the air, and that promotes oxygenation of your cells. Nasal breathing through the night cleans and keeps the sinus clear. If you're breathing through your mouth at night, chances are you wake up with a sore, dry throat or stuffy nose—all the more reason to tape your mouth shut.

It also provided some comic relief in my marriage. Once the tape is on, my husband loves to ask me questions that are more than a yes or no answer. We've taken pantomime to a whole new level.

## PUTTING IT ALL TO BED

Sleep might be the most important thing you do for your brain and body, after breathing, of course. You can go for a few days without food and water, even sleep. But your health can become a nightmare without the sleep you need.

*When I wake up, I am reborn.*
—MAHATMA GANDHI

### CHAPTER SUMMARY

☑ A good night's sleep is as important to your health as diet and exercise, possibly even more important.

☑ Keep a consistent schedule for bedtime and waking. To get the most out of a good night sleep, if possible, wake without an alarm.

☑ Be smart about what you eat and drink, especially close to bedtime. Keep big meals, caffeine, and alcohol to a minimum.

☑ Control your room environment and temperature. Get comfy with a good quality mattress, sheets, pillow, and pajamas, and create a sleep sanctuary in the bedroom. Keep the bedroom cool and dark.

☑ Have a relaxing bedtime ritual. Wind down and clear your head with breathing exercises or meditation before bed.

☑ Consider using an eye wrap, earplugs and cloth tape over the center of your mouth to improve nasal breathing.

## CHAPTER EIGHT

# Sex Is Part of Nature, I Go with Nature

*But as for you, be fruitful and multiply; spread out across the earth and multiply upon it.*
—THE BOOK OF GENESIS 9:7

Maslow's hierarchy of needs has sex as the last physiological need for the survival of mankind. We needed to have sex. The male sperm needs to wiggle its way into a woman's egg, mixing up two sets of DNA to successfully make more of us, so the human species will carry on. Big yeah!

Marilyn Monroe famously said, "Sex is part of nature, I go along with nature."

I plan to prove Maslow and Marilyn wrong.

It was 1943 when Maslow published his hierarchy of needs theory. That was a time when World War II was coming to an end. Women were marrying a little younger, around age twenty instead of twenty-two. The GI Bill of Rights made home purchases more affordable for veterans. Jobs were plentiful. The American Dream of having a family, home, and way to pay for it all was a reality. All this started the beginning of one of the biggest baby booms in United States history.

Marriages had been put off during the war years. The world was unsafe, men were off fighting, and women were doing their part working jobs at home to support the war. With the war over, young couples wanted to marry and start families, and apparently the old-fashioned way of making a baby through sex was working pretty well. From 1944 to 1961, birth rates soared with more than sixty-five million children born during this time, creating the generation known as baby boomers.

Suburbs sprung up as an economic and community-oriented way to raise the new fast-multiplying brood. Resources seemed plentiful, government and public opinion supported women staying home to raise their children, and life seemed pretty darn good. With the drudgery of war over, families settled into the suburbs, new products were developed to meet consumer needs, and everything seemed hunky-dory.[50]

For a while, anyway.

Life did move on post-war, but around twenty-five years later, birth rates plummeted to their lowest since World War II ended. What happened?

During those postwar decades, conservative attitudes dramatically changed. The baby boomers grew up, and had very different ideas on marriage, especially the part about having children and sex. The sexual revolution of the later decades was the cat out of the bag—but before we get to that we need to back up to before Victorian era prudishness,

For centuries, a Victorian moral code of abstinence, with a threat of hellfire and damnation if broken, provided a successful deterrent for most promiscuous behavior outside of marriage.

Morality and sexuality were linked, and the Christian doctrine associated the godliest life with abstinence. Sex was allowed only within the confines of marriage and for the purpose of reproduction. Contraception was banned because that meant the possibility of sex for pleasure instead of procreation. The other threat was contraception would limit child births. Limiting children was against most religious doctrine as the best way to increase the number of any society was to create more people through increased births.

For many men and women suffering through the horrors of World War II, thinking about your eternal life and possible damnation was unimportant when your daily life was already hell. But the Victorian attitudes did carry over to those men and women. In the post-war era, the only socially acceptable thing to do for regular access to sex was to marry.

**No matter how much cats fight,**
**there always seem to be plenty of kittens.**
—ABRAHAM LINCOLN

# FOR ENTERTAINMENT PURPOSES ONLY

The crack in sexual attitudes started to show when the *Kinsey Report*s were published in 1948 and 1953. The report found alarmingly high statistics on men who visited prostitutes and had extramarital affairs, and both men and women who had homosexual experiences. The time was ripe to toss out Victorian prudishness for the new sexual revolution.

Sex was no longer a marriage-oriented project but more about discovering one's own pleasures. The Christian belief that sex was somehow wrong because it was pleasurable quickly lost out. Probably because sex was very pleasurable, and by the skyrocketing birth rates of the boomer days, couples were having loads of sex.

The crack widened in 1953 when Hugh Hefner founded *Playboy* magazine, the first men's magazine to feature nude women and articles fueling sexual liberation. The first issue sold over fifty thousand copies and featured none other than Marilyn Monroe on the cover.

The crack split wide open in the 1960s, the decade of the all-out sexual revolution. The first oral contraceptive was approved by the US Food and Drug Administration, and that was it—the crack turned into an avalanche snowballing unstoppably forward.

It all culminated in the 1970s, the decade of free love. Although birth control pills had been approved by the FDA in the 1960s, it wasn't until 1972 that the Supreme Court legalized birth control for all women, irrespective of marital status.[51] In 1973, with the judgment of Roe v. Wade, the Supreme Court legalized birth control through abortion. Sex without childbirth was available either way, from a proactive or reactive stance. Childbirth could be eliminated as a possible outcome from a sexual encounter. In heterosexual relationships, women were liberated, and men were possibly happier for it.

All this only proves sex was eventually legitimized for pleasure, and not just for procreation. In fact, I would venture to say most sex happening around the world today is not for reproduction. When the fear of conception is subtracted, what's left has proven to be more than just pleasure. It's the connection between those who are having sex. You get pleasure from the relationship, as well as the sex. If it were only sexual pleasure or release, masturbation would do the trick. We're different from most other animals in that we not only seek pleasure from sex, we also love to give pleasure through sex. It's the ebb and flow of giving and receiving that sets us apart.

Pleasure, whether sexual or otherwise, is part of our human make up. We gravitate to pure pleasure to survive, but sleep could be at the top of your pleasure list instead of sexual desire. Pleasure comes in many varieties, and sex is just one flavor.

The coming of age for the baby boomers happened during the sexual revolution of the sixties and decade of free love in the seventies. They grew up into adults, and when they started families, it was on their own terms, selecting whether and when to have children. In the meantime, there was still sex.

> **Love is the answer, but while you are waiting for the answer, sex raises some pretty good questions.**
>
> —WOODY ALLEN

Maslow was now half wrong.

Sex for pleasure may not be strong enough to be on the list of survival needs. The other physiological needs deal with life-or-death issues, like hunger or being too cold. You're not going to die without sex. Maslow's 1943 view of sex may be outdated now, but there's still the issue of procreation. Do we need sex to procreate and keep the species going?

July 1978, in Oldham, England, Louise Brown was born. She was the first baby ever born through in vitro fertilization, or IVF. IVF is a process of fertilization that combines the egg and sperm outside the woman's body in a laboratory. Today, you can store nonfertilized eggs, sperm, or the fertilized embryos for future use. The options are wide open.

There it is. Maslow was wrong. We don't even need sex for procreation.

## THE TALK

When my nieces and nephew were somewhere around high school age, they got "the talk." Not the sex talk from Mom or Dad about the birds and the bees, but the talk from me, Auntie Cindy.

Aunt Cindy's talk became a good source of banter among the cousins. They asked each other if they had gotten "the talk." Who had gotten "the talk," who hadn't, and when they could expect it.

There was a wink and a chuckle from those who had, and looks of confusion and terror from those who hadn't.

The talk was a deal consisting of three promises I asked them to make. The deal and the three promises involved what they would be doing with their life by the age of twenty-five.

1. That by the age of twenty-five, they would be contributing members of society.
2. That they didn't get married until they were twenty-five.
3. That they didn't have any babies until after they were married.

Number one was a two-part promise.

One, that they had their education in order, whether that meant high school, college, graduate school, trade school, or an apprenticeship.

Two, that they had employment and weren't just sitting in their parents' basement watching TV, playing video games or picking lint out of their navel. That they were contributing members of society in whatever ways they choose. That they were involved in church, sports, activities or other groups that supported a community spirit. In essence, they needed to develop their own rich life.

Numbers two and three are pretty clear.

If they kept all these promises, the big reward would be that I would put them in my will and grant them a portion of my estate. Plus, there were more immediate perks of vacations, events, and experiences.

When appropriate, I would help them with their financial decisions and, most importantly, helped them buy a house so they could live mortgage-free. My nephew had the best witty response. He wanted to know if we're talking about a, five-, six-,or God willing—seven-figure number.

There's a reason I choose the age of twenty-five as a dividing line for them. A consensus of neuroscientists determined that the brain may not fully develop until the midtwenties. But eighteen is the legal age in the United States for consenting to massive student debt, marriage, or military service. These adult decisions are being made by a brain that most likely is not fully developed. Heck, the legal age for alcohol is twenty-one, so that says a lot. These young adults are more likely to engage in riskier choices. The immature brain lacks the developmental skills for decision-making, impulse control, logical thinking, complex planning, risk management, and attention span.[52]

The three promises focused on two critical goals in a person's life: career and family. My goal was to establish the age of twenty-five as a marker, and I gave them the neuroscientific reasons why. Some young adults mature faster than others, but age twenty-five and the three promises was something they could easily remember.

They all made good decisions and that's all I could ask. Like them, it's important to consider how and when you make decisions, especially when it comes to the responsibility—particularly with sex.

*If you want to make God laugh, tell him about your plans.*
−WOODY ALLEN

## WHAT'S THE PLAN?

As we said at the beginning of the book, a mistake is an action or judgment that's misguided or wrong. When you're continuing to make the same mistakes over and over, that becomes your decision. Own it. When it comes to sex, there's one decision above all others. You have to have a plan and stick to it, even in the heat of the moment.

When a man and a woman engage in sex without taking effective birth control measures, you are both taking a considerable risk that the woman may wind up pregnant. Then what?

It's okay when adults make poor decisions that affect the trajectory of their own lives, but now you have involved an innocent party—the baby.

I have people in my life who are the product of an unplanned pregnancy. Their parents were single at the time of conception, but that quickly changed with a hastily planned wedding. I also have other very close friends who are adopted. I'm blessed to have them all in my life, and am deeply grateful their mothers made the choice to continue the pregnancy, have the baby, and then give the baby up.

The Guttmacher Institute, which reports on abortion trends, found that in 1972, 16 pregnancies per 1,000 were terminated. Abortion trends peaked around 1980 with 29 per 1,000 pregnancies terminated. As of 2014, 14 per 1,000 pregnancies were terminated or over 926,200 abortions compared to 4,090,000 live births for the same year.[53] That means about 18 percent of pregnancies were terminated. That's a significant number for something wholly preventable.

Sixty-two percent of reproductive-age women are currently using some form of birth control.[54] Remember, it's a choice to make now. Plan and protect yourself from unwanted pregnancies or be prepared for the consequences.

## SEX IN PART OF NATURE

As for Marilyn's statement, "Sex is part of nature, I go along with nature." Okay, I have to agree, Marilyn was right and I was wrong.

In nature, sex is everywhere. All the multicellular creatures on earth reproduce in some way. All sexual reproduction has two members of a species somehow combining their DNA to produce offspring.

The instinctual sex drive is so strong in some species, it even drives them to decorate.

In the forests of Australia and parts of New Guinea, there's a crazy little bird that goes to great lengths to lure a mate. The male bowerbird builds a very elaborate display area or bower—thus the name. It's usually made up of twigs set up on end, creating a sort of open-air hut, and contains stolen trinkets, perhaps stolen from unsuspecting picnic-goers in the area or other male bowerbirds' nests.

The male bowerbird is meticulous. The bower is his dance floor for his impressive mating ritual dance. Should a female enter the bower area, the male starts his elaborate dance. A waving of the wings and she is mesmerized. Her pupils recede to pinpoints, indicating her attention is transfixed and for the male to proceed. The ritual continues with more moves, strutting his stuff until the female succumbs or flies off, uninterested. The ritual varies among each variety of bower bird, but overall, their complex mating behavior may be the most elaborate of all birds.

Humans go through rituals as well to make themselves appealing in the hopes of a sexual encounter. Early man might have killed a gazelle and dragged it into the cave, but today's man, and woman, have a few more choices. Beauty may be in the eye of the beholder but with over eighteen billion dollars a year being spent on deodorant and antiperspirants, how you smell might be a close second to how you look.[55]

Being appealing today takes work but there are a here are a few winning tips:

1. Use your captivating smile. Nothing says, "hello there" more than an engaging smile.
2. Show confidence. Strut your stuff—strutting starts with good posture. Fitness and good posture go a long way to building confidence.

3. Keep your personal hygiene up—your hair, facial hair, hands and nails be well-kept.
4. Have a sense of style with flattering clothes.
5. Always be polite. Be positive. Have a sense of humor.
6. Be attentive and listen. Also, have a few good stories ready to tell of your own,

At times, the human sex drive, or libido, may cause us to do crazy things. Like the bowerbird, both men and women can go to great lengths to make themselves more appealing by changing behavior, dress, appearances, and activities. We put ourselves out there in hopes of making a connection, but there are ground rules for all sexual encounters, whether love based or for pleasure sake.

## RULES OF ENGAGEMENT

For starters, you have to be of legal age and give full consent for any sexual encounter. Then use precautions to eliminate the risk of sexually transmitted diseases. If pregnancy is not wanted, use effective birth control. Sharing your body with someone is an intimate act. In this equation, you're literally giving part of yourself to someone. Make sure they're worth it. After that, have a good time. After all, sex is part of our primal instincts and a pleasurable act.

A normal, healthy sex drive is whatever someone is comfortable with. In other words, normal doesn't exist. The bottom line is we're all just people wanting connection with a caring person, as well as love, pleasure, and a good life.

When drinking, doing drugs or being otherwise impaired, people often make poor choices. The regrettable tattoo, driving a car under the influence, or entering into a sexual encounter that otherwise probably wouldn't have happened. Alcohol can lower your inhibitions and make you feel more confident and sexier, or less inhibited. There's a point, however, when lowered inhibitions escalate to being out of control. If you're the one who's out of control, you're not in a position to be making any big decisions, other than deciding it's probably time to go home. Drunken sex and consent can be an impossible mix.

Sexual advances can sometimes be hard to read, whether you're drinking or sober. We give off vibes we're open to advances or flirtations to let someone know we are interested in them. Sexual encounters and advances sometimes happen with implied consent, meaning people give and are attempting to read those vibes. Sexual advances are not always a specific ask-and-response situation—you're not announcing your next move and getting explicit affirmation to proceed. Often, the participants just go with the flow. Consent can be a fluid concept, but there are rules. No, means no. Stop, means stop. And anyone who is impaired is incapable of giving consent, implied or explicit, and the assumption needs to be a very firm *no*.

With sexual intimacy you're inviting a person into your most sacred space. Consensual sex, intimacy or touching between persons is the mutual transgression of physical boundaries. Both parties need to feel secure, be without doubts, be of sound mind, and remain unimpaired by drugs or alcohol. Consent must be explicit and clear. Yes means an agreement to engage in sexual activity without abuse or exploitation of—in legal terms— "trust, power or authority," coercion or threats, and it can be revoked at any time, even during the act itself. Again, no, means no to anything and everything. No means stop, *now*.

## IN THE MOOD FOR LOVE

There are two ways we get in the mood, for love, turned on and ready to get down.

One is through spontaneous desire that happens when a mental interest in sex pops up. Out of the blue, you find yourself thinking about sex and want to have it. According to sex educator Emily Nagoski about 75 percent of men and about 15 percent of women experience spontaneous desire.

The other way we get in the mood for sex is through responsive desire. It usually happens when you're already having a physical stimulating experience like kissing. You didn't start out in the mood for sex, but one thing led to another, and the next thing you know your naked and doing it.[56]

In a TED Talk, Emily Nagoski explains some common qualities of couples who sustain a good sexual connection. She points out that most couples who have been together for decades are not having sex often or are sexually wild and adventurous. They're very busy people with careers, often kids, and other outside commitments that, like everything in life, create a huge time suck. In fact, the strongest predictors of a healthy relationship and sexual satisfaction had nothing to do with what kind of sex or how wild or often, but it was all about whether they cuddled after sex.[57]

Emily goes on to reveal two commonalities among couples with healthy sexual connections:

First, that they have a strong friendship, specifically strong trust. That they are emotionally present and available to each other.

Second, that they prioritize sex. Sex is not an afterthought. These couples put aside everything else on the endless to-do list, even sleep, and create a space where all they're going to do is touch skin to skin and see how it progresses.

Sex may not be on the list of our survival needs as Maslow first hypothesized. It's an important part of our primal instincts, and it could contribute more to a meaningful part of any partner-committed relationship. And for most, it's just plain fun.

## ONE-NIGHT STANDS

As long as both parties are on the same page, sex can be for enjoyment. It's not meaningless sex, exactly. It's more something that just feels nice. Using each other for sex doesn't make it empty, it just makes it not serious. Not everything has to be fraught with a future. It may be just right—for now.

Where's this one-night stand going? Nowhere, and that can be fine.

Sex doesn't hurt people. People hurt people. One-night stands do have meaning. They mean you want to enjoy sex.

*If passion drives you, let reason hold the reins.*
—BENJAMIN FRANKLIN

---

### CHAPTER SUMMARY

☑  Sex is an intimate, personal arrangement between people.

☑  Remember: people hurt people.

☑  Love and sex are sometimes two separate things.

☑  Have a plan for sex. If you don't want pregnancy, don't have sex, or don't have sex without effective birth control. By the way, the only 100 percent effective birth control is abstinence.

---

# PART TWO

---

# On the Outside

*The environment is everything that isn't me.*
—ALBERT EINSTEIN

*When you know nature as part of yourself, you will act in harmony. When you feel yourself part of nature, you will live in harmony.*
—TAO TE CHING

## THE ENVELOPE WE LIVE IN

Our environment is everything that is outside of and around us. Air, whether it's the crisp air of an Alpine meadow or the toxic gases of bulging factory smoke, our body depends on the health of our surroundings to sustain the health of our bodies.

After the health of our body, which is totally dependent on our environment, our environment itself can be supportive and nurturing for our spirit or damaging causing undue stress, anxiety or pain.

In a study, Bruce Alexander, a researcher from Simon Fraser University, separated rats into two different cages. One cage was an isolated, small cage with nothing in it. The other cage was roomy, full of stimulating things to do and loads of other rats to have fun with. Both cages were equipped with two water bottles to drink from, one with regular water and the other water laced with morphine. The isolated rats quickly became addicted to the morphine laced water. The stimulated rats almost never touched the morphine laced water. The conclusion was the environment was more of a contributing factor in drug addiction than what we previously thought.[58]

In this section, we go outside the body needs to discover how we depend on and interact with our environment. We'll discover how the environment, along with other people, places and things in our environment truly affect the course and happiness of our lives.

CHAPTER NINE

# Making Sense of The World

**You carry Mother Earth within you. She is not outside of you. Mother Earth is not just your environment. In that insight of inter-being it is possible to have real communication with the Earth, which is the highest form of prayer.**

—THICK NHAT HANH, BUDDHIST MONK

In Part One: On the Inside, we identified the things that affect our body's physiological needs. In Part Two: On the Outside, we move into Maslow's second level, Safety. It's concerned with everything outside our body and the physical environment we live in. To survive, we need to live in a harmonious symbiotic relationship with our environment.

First, we look to our environment to supply us with the necessities to keep our bodies alive; we need sustenance like food, water, and clean air to breathe. Millenia ago, people built dwellings around freshwater and fertile soil. Today, we have water treatment plants and food delivered globally. Our needs remain the same, but the supply chain has exponentially expanded.

Second, we need protection from the harsh elements of our environment. For shelter, we've gone from caves to condos. For protecting our bodies, we've gone from animal skins to breathable fabrics. We've developed air-conditioning, air fresheners, sunscreens, bug repellents, moisturizers, and other creature comforts, making our existence in the world wonderful. Chopping and storing enough wood to last the winter has been replaced with flipping a switch to power our HVAC system to the desired temperature.

Our environment is our envelope of living and has the most significant impact on our comfort, protection, and survival. Also, it's one of the biggest reasons for our technological advancements. We like to be pampered and what better way to do that than invent stuff we didn't know we needed? As an example, the Snuggie, a blanket you can wear, has sold over thirty million products, making five hundred million dollars.

Third, we need other animals: oxen to plow fields, cows for meat and dairy, horses to aid in travel, and dogs for companionship. Plows have been replaced with combines. Meat can be grown in labs, horses have been replaced with crossover SUV's, but thank God, we still need dogs.

Fourth, we need protection from things that will do us harm, like other animals that would like to eat us. Most of our likely predators have been caged in zoos or banished to game preserves on the African savannas. However, we still need protection from a different kind of predator— cybercriminals stealing our identity, people out to take our money or rob us of our property, or companies that put profit before public safety.

Fifth, we need laws to govern us, protect us, and allow us to move freely in society without fear of undue restraint or false imprisonment. We have civil rights that include certain rights—to vote, to a fair trial, to government services, to public education, and to use public facilities. We have seat belt safety laws and laws against discrimination. All these rights, regulations, and laws are to protect our liberties and provide equal treatment.

Here's where your eighth-grade American history class will come in handy. Before the United States of America became a sovereign country on July 4, 1776, the individual states were colonies of the British Empire. The collection of colonies was referred to as the United Colonies or the British Colonies. The king and the Parliament of Great Britain ruled the colonies and had imposed heavy taxes on the colonists, but the colonists had no representation in the British government. That, other unfair treatment, and egregious acts pushed the colonists to revolt.

On March 23, 1775, Henry James presented a proposal to the Second Virginia Convention at Richmond. The meeting was held at St. John's Church in secrecy so the British wouldn't know. England had not responded to the colonists' latest proposition for reconciliation, and Henry James proposed the colonists should ready themselves for the possibility of revolution—of war. That they needed to organize a volunteer militia in each county of Virginia to be ready to defend the area should England not accept the terms and begin military action against them.

The presentation by Henry James was not officially transcribed, but everyone remembered his closing words, "Give me liberty or give me death."

James had so eloquently put into words just how far the new colonists were willing to take their pursuit of freedom—to the death.

That's how strongly we feel for all our civil liberties, our laws established for the good of the community, the protection of the people, and the freedom of action and speech.

The First Amendment to the Constitution protects each citizen's five fundamental freedoms: freedom of religious pursuits, freedom of speech, freedom of the press, freedom to assemble and freedom to petition the government to change. These civil liberties are the cornerstone of our democracy. As the colonists sought to protect themselves from the tyranny of British rule, civil liberties protect us from government power.

All five elements highlight how interdependent we must be with our natural environment, animals, other people, communities, nations and everything on our planet. The need to live harmoniously and in symbiosis with our environment and other people or nations remains the same. The threats to our existence have simply upgraded from lions chasing us to having to install malware on our computers to protect us from cyberattacks.

## BIG CLAWS OR BIG BRAINS

Early man was an unlikely candidate for becoming the dominant species compared to animals that were faster, stronger, and had bigger teeth and claws. But we had the advantage: for our size, we had bigger, more complex brains. To evolve, you can become stronger like those animals with big teeth and claws, or you can become smarter, as man did.

As our brains grew more complex, our cognitive abilities grew as well and helped us make tools and weapons to protect ourselves from the predators with big teeth. We could think, adapt, and innovate. As part of those innovations, we learned to cook our food. Cooking food helps denature proteins and remove harmful bacteria. It softens foods and makes nutrients easily absorbable. We also learned to build shelters to protect ourselves.

Over time, we developed a culture of social learning, passing down from generation to generation skills like toolmaking, language, innovations, and creativity. We formed groups to share the workload, which led to a higher chance of survival, success in reproduction, and increasing the tribe's numbers. The bigger the tribe, the bigger the chance of survival.

In our modern daily life, we don't encounter many animals that are out to eat us. Like our ancestors, we still have an ingrained awareness of things that could kill us or do us harm. We have a natural aversion to snakes because many of them are poisonous, and a snake's bite is very unpleasant. We have an instinctual drive to protect our body from the elements, through wrapping ourselves in fur pelts has been replaced by manufacturing warm, waterproof clothes. We've built condos and houses to live in and grocery stores to forage in. We don't have to hunt down a gazelle—our meats come neatly packed in plastic wrap to avoid bacterial contamination.

The same needs for safety drive modern man. Most products we buy today need to be safe and effective. They need to be useful, solve problems, and protect us from potential threats, no matter how great or small.

For example, the Food and Drug Administration (FDA) is set-up to review and approve medications that will improve our lives, manage diseases, and help us live longer. The FDA is responsible for the protection of public health by ensuring the safety and efficacy of those medications.

Another example: Playtex developed plastic gloves, the Playtex Living Gloves, to protect our hands when we wash dishes. When buying a car, we review the safety standards, how many airbags it has, and how the car fared in crash tests compared to other similar models.

In today's world, practically everything we buy is for the comfort or sustainability of our bodies in the world. The needs of modern man and early man are the same. The environment and our choices are now a lot snazzier all because of our big brains and cognitive development.

## WOOLY MAMMOTH ON THE FREEWAY

Our need for safety dominates our behavior and is driven by our senses: sight, smell, touch, taste, and hearing. Our senses are our internal early warning and a GPS system. Early man would see a bush rustle or hear a noise, and his senses would go on high alert. Could it be a hungry saber-tooth tiger? Is there a danger?

*When all is said and done, we only exist in relation to the world, and our senses evolved as scouts who work together to bridge that divide and provide volumes of information, warnings, and rewards.*

—DIANE ACKERMAN, AMERICAN POET AND NATURALIST

It's the fight-or-flight response mode that warns us and supplies us with environmental information to determine friend or foe, danger or not. If we're safe, we stay. If unsafe, we leave (i.e., flight) or attempt to change the situation by becoming the aggressor (i.e., fight).[59] We are no different from early man. Even if the stakes are not life-threatening, we still have the same innate drive to fight or flee if a situation seems in any way harmful.

Like a wooly mammoth barging through the bushes, a car merging into our lane of traffic is perceived as a similar high-level threat. The fight-or-flight mode kicks in, and we either get the hell out of the way (flight) or honk our horn (fight). This emotional avalanche of fear shoots adrenaline into the bloodstream, increases our heart rate, and shunts blood away from our extremities to the essential organs. Even though a car merging into our lane is typically not life-threatening, our body reacts as if it's the wooly mammoth out to run us down.

The body goes into DEFCON—emergency lockdown, and its chain reaction is the same whether it is a perceived high-level threat or an actual high-level threat. Evolution has not synced our outdated fight-or-flight mode to the experiences of our modern world.

*Actual threats* endanger our existence or are life-threatening. They're real.

*Perceived threats* initiate unwarranted anxieties. They're situations that are perceived as endangering to our existence but are not. Our body reacts as strongly as if they are our actual threat.

Our fight-or-flight mode is programmed into our genes and is very useful if, say, you're a soldier fighting a battle. When out on patrol, soldiers are on high-alert, scanning the area for dangers and performing their duties.

Today's fast-paced, stressful world may seem like a battlefield to the average person's fight-or-flight mode. Acute, quick actions prompted by sudden excessive levels of stress can save our lives when necessary, but chronic stress can do the opposite. A state of chronic stress can lead to many serious health issues, including depression, anxiety, cardiovascular disease, high blood pressure, heart arrhythmias, heart attacks, and stroke.

Today, the stakes are very different, and our primal instincts may be getting the better of us. At work, maybe you were overlooked for the promotion you were expecting. You believe your financial future and livelihood is threatened. Your hot head takes over, and you storm into your boss's office to yell in his face—fight—or run from the office in tears heading for the nearest bar—flight.

Maybe you do neither, but you sure wanted to. You thought about it. Our reaction, whether we act on it or not, is still happening in the body. The body goes into DEFCON with the racing heart, skyrocketing adrenaline levels, and blood shunts from our extremities in an effort to protect our vital organs, all creating high levels of stress and anxiety.

Our survival needs are no longer running from the raging, wooly mammoth but running to meet deadlines at work. Money, work, job stability, the economy, family responsibilities, personal health, and law and order are the new standards for Maslow's second level. They all relate to our survival. We don't sleep in caves, but we buy three-bedroom houses in the suburbs. We need to make sure our physical well-being is protected. Doing that in today's world is a constant battle that overloads our senses, ultra-stressing our system.

*Every second of every day, our senses bring in way too much data than we can possibly process in our brains.*
—PETER DIAMANDIS, FOUNDER OF THE X PRIZE FOUNDATION

In the 1980s, cell phones started to populate our lives. But with today's smartphones, our nine-to-five work life has become a 24/7 all-consuming need to respond. This constant source of stress initiates the same response as a real threat would. That's what we're doing with our days—dealing with perceived threats and in turn, the fear and anxiety they create.

The world is a hectic place, and the struggles of juggling work, careers, and home life can create chronic stress, anxiety, and depression that becomes debilitating. Reported by the Anxiety and Depression Association of America, anxiety disorders are the most common mental illness in the United States, affecting approximately forty million adults or over 18 percent of the population. Further, only 40 percent of those suffering from anxiety receive treatment, and nearly half of those diagnosed with depression are also suffering from anxiety.[60]

## FUTURE SHOCK

For several million years, the human brain continuously scanned the horizon for threats it needed to avoid. We sensed changes in light, sounds, temperature, and everything else in our environment. In ancestral man's dangerous world, we sought out food and shelter, and the use of senses helped with those tasks.

In today's world, the brain has adapted to be able to perceive dangers in the far future. We're no longer just looking to kill a gazelle for the day's meal. We've created future threats. Where would we be without health insurance, dental floss, or the 401(k) plan? These are all responses to perceived threats that loom in our distant future, but that we deal with today.

We can spend far too much time in the anxiety or defensive mode. Every uncomfortable text or Facebook post sets off a threat response in your system. We respond, and our body locks up in survival mode. Even when we have no visual cue or firsthand experience with an actual threat, we can exaggerate the risks as if it were about to happen in real time. No matter how irrational, we can elevate an unlikely threat as if it were an immediate or actual threat.

## SHARK ATTACK

I am a surfer. Out in the ocean off Santa Monica, California, where Sunset Boulevard dead-ends into the Pacific Coast Highway is my favorite place to catch waves. North of there is a breeding ground for sharks. According to Chris Lowe, professor of marine biology at Cal State Long Beach, "Most people do not realize that our front yard—L.A.'s front yard—is home to one of the largest nurseries for white sharks in the world." At birth, white sharks measure five feet and are immediately on their own hunting for food. The shallow waters off the California coast provide protection from predators, like other bigger sharks and killer whales, and the juveniles have plenty of stingrays and fish to eat in these shallows.[61]

As a surfer, I'm aware of this fact. I know a five-footer could chomp off my leg, and I can live with that truth. Last week, I saw an eight-footer breaching about fifty yards out off the nose of my surfboard. After years in the water, I don't stress about it. I am not crazy, although all my friends think I am.

I have friends who wouldn't set a toe in the ocean for their fear of being attacked by a shark. Everyone who knows I surf thinks I'm crazy for putting my life in danger. If I had a dollar for every time I was asked about sharks, I could turn in my surfboard for a boat. My friends' perception of threat far outweighs the reality of the danger. According to Wikipedia's,

"List of fatal shark attacks in California," since 1980, there have been ... guess how many? Got a number? It's only nine. The risk of a fatal car crash outweighs a deadly shark attack by a long shot. In 2017, California had 3,602 fatal car crashes, second to Texas with 3,702.[62]

Our irrational fear of sharks is more about our emotional response than reality. We're afraid of losing control, of the unfamiliar, and of things or situations not being predictable. "While we can sense fear, and we can interpret fear, the actual feeling of fear is completely outside of our control," says Blake Chapman, author of Shark Attacks: *Myths, Misunderstandings, and Human Fear*. Our feelings of fear happen more often than the reality of the actual threat.

Unfamiliar risks are perceived as higher than they are. The risk of terrorism causes far more anxiety than common street crime, even though the latter claims many more lives. People fear their children will be given poisoned candy by strangers at Halloween, even though there has been no documented case of this ever happening.[63]

Our human brain oversimplifies numbers too. The statistic of your chance of being killed by a shark is 1 in 3,748,067. That number is way too abstract for the brain to comprehend. You're more likely to die by a dog attack, lightning strike or car crash.[64] It may be irrelevant that shark attacks are extremely rare. Statistically unfounded, but we have a disproportionate level of distress, worry, and fear over an emotional trigger—the shark.

Sharks are not alone. We have the same disproportionate fear over many situations in our life that are even more relevant. We can worry about the simplest things.

> *My life has been filled with terrible misfortune;*
> *most of which never happened.*
> —MICHEL DE MONTAIGNE, FRENCH RENAISSANCE PHILOSOPHER

Maslow's second level, Safety, is about how we deal with the struggles of existence in our environment. We have a life with physiology, and now we need to protect, nurture, and enhance that life through living in our environment. We need housing, food, protection for our body, and the means to pay for it all in our complex modern world. We need employment. For our survival and well-being, we need sustained employment through job security, laws and order to protect us, seat belts to reduce fatal car crashes, sanitation projects to protect our drinking water, and then there's everything else in our environment we need to survive. Every environmental hiccup can exert an effect on our existence. At times, it's a lot to handle.

It's why humans love predictability. We love certainty and avoid uncertainty like the plague.

For most, the threat of uncertainty generates a strong threat response in our limbic system. Like an addiction to anything, when the craving for certainty is met, there is a sensation of reward. Repeating patterns give us pleasure as they meet our expectations and earlier predictions.[65] We feel more in control when things go the way we thought they would. We feel more comfortable when we know what a future event will be like and what will happen. We have restaurants we know are good and grocery stores that carry our brand of products. We map out routes for our commute that take a predictable amount of time for our commute, and when that predictability is interrupted by a fender-bender, we go into a state of stress.

When things go awry, our fear bubbles up.

> *If you are depressed, you are living in the past.*
> *If you are anxious, you are living in the future.*
> *If you are at peace, you are living in the present.*
>
> —LAO TZU

# FIFTY-FIFTY RULE

Anxiety and stress over what will or will not happen is mental noise. Mental noise is like trying to do calculus in a handstand, while acid rock music is playing loud enough to make your ears bleed. Okay, I'm exaggerating, but mental noise is anxiety on overload. We source our past experiences, bringing up stress and regret, and often apply them to future events. Is what you're fretting over likely to happen or not? There is a difference between possibility, however remote, and probability. We most often fret over the unlikely possibilities.

Worry, doubts, and anxieties are all part of life's journey. Still, when your brain is looping in circles faster than a NASCAR race, your worries magnify the situation well beyond the limits of reality. Then, it's time to worry about your worrying. If you're paralyzed over your upcoming root canal, global warming, the fate of fruit flies, or whether alien life forms will like Beethoven's Fifth Symphony put in the *Voyager* spacecraft destined to travel forty thousand years into the future, then it's time to wean yourself off worrying.

> **The greatest weapon against stress is our ability to choose one thought over another.**
> – WILLIAM JAMES, AMERICAN PHILOSOPHER

Worrying doesn't change a damn thing. When you're overwhelmed, frayed about future issues, or feeling paralyzed about potential problems, put it to my fifty-fifty rule: It will or it won't. Meaning everything will work out—but if it doesn't, then it won't.

Looking to the future is a necessary means to make rational decisions, learn, grow, develop, and plan. Set a plan. Then know things happen that might derail that plan, and that's just the way it goes. Life is full of stressful situations. Dwelling on all the negative crap that could happen can paralyze you. Could've, should've, would've, are all useless.

When you surrender to the fifty-fifty rule, where everything becomes it will or it won't, life becomes a little simpler. You can't control time. We all get the same twenty-four-hour day. Letting needless worry deduct minutes or hours from your day is a choice.

**_Adventure is just bad planning._**
—ROALD AMUNDSEN, NORWEGIAN EXPLORER OF THE ANTARCTIC

## MASTER OF MINDFULNESS

Most of our lives are spent focused on doing stuff around us. Things happen, and we react. Mindfulness is to bring awareness to what our minds and bodies are doing.

Buddha told a story to enlighten the practice and explain how it works for the mind.

One day, there was Mr. Turtle and Mr. Fox, who accidentally met in the forest. The fox thought the turtle would make a good meal. The turtle thought, Oh no, the fox is going to eat me. He's my enemy. I can't run. I'm not fast enough to get away. Instead, the turtle went inside his shell. The fox waited, poking around the turtle's shell, but got tired and went away.

The fox in our lives is stress, tension, anxiety, sadness, and worry. Be more like the turtle and retreat to your shell. Observe your reaction to the problems at hand, not engaging but appreciating that these feelings, as uncomfortable as they are, will pass, if you let your mind do so.

In stressful situations, you don't need to fight, surrender to the problem, or run away. You can make friends with your problems. You can bring the quality of mindfulness to anything you do during your day. No matter how mundane or stressful, bringing your mindfulness to the situation may help your brain accept where you are. Difficulties will happen, stress is inevitable, but it's your choice how to deal with it. You can let it consume you, or just observe it and know your reaction to stress will most likely pass with time.

For beginners in meditation, the nature of the mind is to time travel. We look backward, ruminating about past experiences, or have anxiety, calling up memories, regrets, or fears. Our mind can even race with thoughts. This is called the monkey mind. Like a monkey swinging from limb to limb, our mind aimlessly wanders. To calm the monkey in you, focus on your breathing patterns. Be kind enough to bring your mind back to your breath. It's the practice of noticing your distraction, and without judgment of yourself, gently bringing your attention back to your breath. The true meaning of mindfulness is to practice being kind to yourself, above all else.

These moments of awakening that light up a portion of the brain are so important. The dorsolateral prefrontal cortex, primarily involved in the management of cognitive processing, is also involved in managing both risky and moral decision-making. Activation can evoke preferences toward equitable options and suppress the temptation of maximizing personal gain. Mental kindness and awareness are what meditation sessions develop.[66]

The quality of paying attention strengthens the practice of creating your own emotional space to deal with disturbing events and help you find a new way to deal with emotions. If you're not happy with yourself on the inside, you won't be happy on the outside. Mindfulness seems to change how we relate to our feelings, which in turn can change how we relate to the world.

# THE EYES ARE THE WINDOW TO THE BRAIN

We hear a loud noise and our attention is immediately diverted to go and investigate what happened. We usually look up when we hear a helicopter passing overhead at a low altitude. It could be the sound of a car crashing or if you have kids, a loud bang inside the house. Especially if you have kids, and with kids, if you don't hear noise, you wonder why and go to investigate what they're up to. Our hearing is only one of our senses that helps us connect with our place in the world.

Through our senses it's our brain's visual processing that's at the forefront. The retina, which contains one hundred and fifty million light-sensitive rod and cone cells, is an outgrowth of the brain. In the brain itself, neurons devoted to visual processing number in the hundreds of millions and take up about 30 percent of the cortex, as compared with 8 percent for touch and just 3 percent for hearing. Each of the two optic nerves, which carry signals from the retina to the brain, consists of a million fibers; each auditory nerve carries a mere thirty thousand.[67]

> *The eye is the most refined of our senses, the*
> *one which communicates most directly*
> *with our mind, our consciousness.*
> —ROBERT DELAUNAY, ARTIST, ORPHIC CUBISM

The brain and eyes act somewhat like a film camera. The cornea is the lens focusing on the image and the iris, much like the aperture of a camera, expands or contracts, allowing levels of light into the eye. But it's the brain that is the digital sensor, recording the images and interpreting their meaning. With more of our neurons dedicated to vision than hearing or sensing touch, vision may be the answer to calming the brain.

> *One touch of nature makes the whole world kin.*
> —WILLIAM SHAKESPEARE, *TROILUS AND CRESSIDA*

# FOREST BATHING

Shinrin-yoku, the art of forest bathing, began in Japan, a country whose urban cities, like Tokyo, are densely populated, but that is two-thirds covered by trees. The belief is there's something special about being in a forest. Qing Li, a Japanese medical doctor and author of *Forest Bathing: How Trees Can Help You Find Health and Happiness*, says, "Let nature enter through your ears, eyes, nose, mouth, hands, and feet." Actively engage your senses to experience the forest.

Japan launched the forest bathing program in 1982. Iiyama, Japan, mainly known for its lush, green forests, has upwards of 2.5 million people walking through those forest trails annually.[68]

The good news about forest bathing is it's a club open to all, and it's free. You and your friends can even start your own Forest Bathing Club with regular scheduled trips to get out into nature.

But what if you can't get to a forest? Would a photo of a forest have some similar visual benefits? We learn and remember best through pictures, not through written or spoken words. Early man learned through what he saw. We're visual people.

So, would seeing a photo of a beautiful mountain setting give our brain a minute of respite?

Leonardo da Vinci wrote that a poet would be overcome by sleep and hunger before being able to describe with words what a painter can depict in an instant.[69] The adage "a picture is worth a thousand words" is sometimes attributed to Napoleon Bonaparte, who said, "A good sketch is better than a long speech." We respond visually. If you can't run off to Japan or elsewhere for a little forest bathing, then pull up a picture on your computer, and visually experience a beautiful setting.

Our visual memory can trigger emotional feelings, so pull up photos of your recent trip to the beach and take a deep breath.

## AWESTRUCK AND ALTRUISM

Since our vision is so essential to our ability to comprehend and process our surroundings, what we see can have an enormous impact on how our brain works. A sense of awe comes when we see and feel the presence of something vast that transcends our understanding of the world.

The Grand Canyon, one of the natural wonders of the world, has been described as awe-inspiring. Standing at the rim of the Grand Canyon, you can look into the vastness of the valley, the copper-colored gorges, and ponder the rock layers that are records of billions of years of history. It's a place of endless wonder that has beckoned exploration. Awe comes in many sizes. The depths of the Grand Canyon and the intricacies of a flower's pistil both can evoke a sense of awe.

Great or small, nature fills our hearts with awe. But we can also feel a sense of awe in response to art, music, poetry, and religious practices. What's happening in the brain when we see something awe-inspiring as opposed to a basket of dirty laundry?

Awe-inspiring moments promote altruism, loving-kindness, and altruistic behavior. When experiencing awe, you're not focused on yourself; your attention shifts to the magnificence outside you. You're not egocentric but seeing a bigger picture. You feel smaller and are more open to prosocial behavior, thinking of the greater good instead of the self. Seeing grandeur is the surprise and reverence. That part of our brain that seeks control and predictability is downgraded, and we become more comfortable with uncertainty or risk, open to a new experience.

*Awe is what moves us forward.*

—JOSEPH CAMPBELL, PROFESSOR OF LITERATURE AT
SARAH LAWRENCE COLLEGE

# HEART IS WHERE THE HOME IS

My niece, Sara, moved to Boulder, Colorado, from Overland Park, Kansas. Her company has a satellite office, so a job was waiting. The primary reason for the move was to live more in nature, to see the mountains every day and spend her weekends hiking trails—sounded good to me. A few weeks after her move, I went to visit to help organize her new apartment.

I'm sort of a visual savant when it comes to furniture, layout, how to place picture frames, and all your interior décor strategies. I have a built-in radar detector for things even slightly askew. My compulsion borders on the need for therapy, but my niece knew I could whip the place together in a weekend—transforming it into her new nest.

As I entered her apartment, my eyes scanned the layout, how she had placed her furniture, and what was on the walls. In the living room was a shelving unit that had a television on the top shelf. Okay—functional. We all need a TV to watch our favorite shows, but from the TV down, the shelves below were barren. To someone who's not a visual savant, that may seem okay, but to me, it wouldn't work at all.

I worked my way around the apartment, moving furniture, adjusting heights of artwork, and making several trips to various retailers for the perfect accessories. We feathered her nest with pillows, curtains, color-coordinated wastebaskets, floor mats, dishes, and bathroom accruements. The empty shelves in the living room were still empty, though. They were haunting me.

As you walked into my niece's apartment, the first thing your eyes would have seen were those empty shelves. Her moving to a new city with no friends or family meant these shelves had to be perfect. They needed to say home. Those empty shelves subconsciously may have triggered thoughts of an empty life. Every time she entered her apartment, that's what she would see, and her subconscious might reverberate that as emptiness. I couldn't take that chance. It had to be perfect. Leaving it for last, I decorated those shelves with meaningful objects from her apartment. The morning I left, I did my final scan before I walked out and felt she was home.

We are visual creatures. I can't say that enough—we take our cues from what we see.

**Set thine house in order.**
—THE BIBLE, 2 KINGS, CHAPTER 20, VERSE 1

# CUES TO THE UNCONSCIOUS MIND

A subliminal message is a technique used in marketing and by advertisers to influence your decision to buy their products. It involves the use of split-second flashes of text, hidden images, and subtle cues that affect the viewer on a level below conscious awareness.

The first reported subliminal ad was from 1947, spotted in a Daffy Duck cartoon on a twirling sign urging viewers to buy war bonds. Since 1958, the technique of subliminal messages by advertisers has been illegal in the United Kingdom, America, and Australia. The European Union banned all tobacco advertising in July 2005, but that didn't stop Marlboro, the cigarette company, from finding another way.

Marlboro was a sponsor of Ferrari, a Formula One car racing team. Formula One is seen by millions all over the world and is a lucrative way to promote a business through sponsoring a car. Marlboro and Ferrari both use a vibrant red for their products, and that similarity made for a good product partnership. But Marlboro had a problem. Because of the ban on cigarette advertising, it could no longer use its logo on the car. Instead, Marlboro opted to stamp a peculiar barcode on the side of the car. At first appearance, it seemed confusing to see a barcode on the side of a Formula One car, but that was the point—it made you look again. The bars' peaks and valleys resembled the word *Marlboro*.[70] This example, and the empty shelves in my niece's apartment, highlight how subliminal messages could be to your disadvantage.

On the harmful side, negative stereotypes and messages we absorb subconsciously throughout our day might sap our inner strength and self-confidence.

In a study, endurance athletes were to exercise on stationary bicycles. They were shown different positive visual cues and subliminal messages like "go," "energy" and happy faces. Others, were shown negative words and unhappy faces. The messages flashed on the screen for less than 0.02 seconds and were mixed in with other content, making the cues unidentifiable to the athletes. When the athlete's got positive visual cues, they were able to go for longer distances and had improved outlooks.

However, your surroundings could be a tool to embed positive messages. Since these cues are working below the threshold of our conscious mind, little things like an organized desk might lead to a more organized day. Inviting bedding might induce restful sleep. Photos of healthy food on the fridge might sway you to eat better. Fresh flowers might evoke a cue of self-love.

We take in our cues visually, and they impact our performance, feelings, attitudes, self-confidence, and mood. Creating a positive environment packed with positive visual cues will reinforce self-esteem and self-confidence.[71]

## A SAFE PLACE TO LAND

Pretend you're moving. That can be frightening. What to pack, toss, donate, bequeath, responsibly recycle, or set on the curb with a sign that says, TAKE ME. It can be cathartic to pretend you're moving and go through the process of elimination on every possession you own. To determine what stays and what goes, ask yourself two very important questions:

Do I love it? Is it useful?

This is an excellent time to say goodbye to cassette tapes unless they're recordings of your grandparent describing what it was like to survive Dachau. Then you may want to take this opportunity to have them digitized for posterity. For everything else, let it be guilt-free, cathartic, and exhilarating to know that in the end, you're left with things that are useful and you love.

When I met my husband, I had a four-bedroom, three-bath beautiful Spanish Colonial home chocked-full of furniture, travel treasures, doo-dads, and tabletop accessories, complete with three sets of china. It may sound like a lifetime of collecting, but I had only lived in the house for only seven years, and most of the home's contents had been purchased during that time. You might have noticed there was a bump in the economy during my nesting phase.

My then boyfriend asked me to marry him. After saying yes, my first thought was, What to do with all my stuff?

My fiancé and I made a pact: we would each get rid of our stuff and come clean to the marriage. We wanted to buy a house that suited both our needs and lifestyles and proceed to fill it with mutually approved stuff. You may have noticed the subsequent bump in the economy during my nesting phase with the new hubby.

As much stuff as I have had and currently possess, it may surprise you to hear I do not consider myself a stuff person. Meaning I have no serious emotional attachment to material objects. Maintaining a guilt-free zone, everything I own has to serve a purpose, and I have to love it.

Along the seven-year nesting period, I had purchased fifty crystal champagne flutes because I found them on sale and hoped to have a gala champagne party ... someday. Someday never came. Now the question was to get rid of them or pack them up and haul them to the new abode. Looking over the champagne flutes, and the other multiples of maybe someday useful objects, put my brain in a frozen state. I felt like I'd been hit by a stun gun. I knew I was overwhelmed, over-matched, and in need of adult supervision, so I called in the professionals. I called my mom.

My mother had always been my Gibraltar, a rock of solid wisdom. She was there to lift me up when I was down, or when too full of myself, to make sure I remembered my humble beginnings. She was my life compass. When I called her to kvetch about my woes, she patiently listened as I listed the overwhelming tasks of dismantling my home. She then espoused this pearl of wisdom that made my brain light up like the caveman who first saw fire.

"You know all the things you bought? You don't own them. They own you."

Wow, why didn't she tell me that before I bought all this stuff, including those champagne flutes? I solved the problem. I had one hell of a garage sale.

When going through your stuff, you might want to keep repeating the mantra:

Do I love it? Is it useful?

It can be a dilemma when faced with Grandma's china that has only three of the needed ten coffee cups for a complete service. Not completely useful, but if you sincerely love the china and the story behind it, get on the Internet and search "replacement china" with the brand name to complete the set and proudly display the china. While you're at it, buy a couple extra coffee cups and plates for the inevitable future breakage. But if you have always disliked pink roses with garish gold trim and resent Grandma for leaving you the incomplete china set instead of her diamond broach, then let it go.

Repeat after me. Do I love it? Is it useful?

When contemplating the usefulness of an object, think of when was the last time you used it, and when you're likely to use it again—daily, yearly, or never in this century? How many pepper mills do you need? More than one on the table and one on the stove? If not, then let it go. When contemplating something you love, what joy does it bring you, and why?

My husband and I have traveled extensively and bought ornaments or little souvenirs along the way that we use to decorate our Christmas tree. We had to switch from a real tree to a reinforced prelit fake tree to support the weight. As soon as it is fully decorated, we circle, head up, head down, scanning the memories of years of travel. Yes, I love it.

> **The objective of cleaning is not just to clean, but to feel happiness living within that environment.**
> —MARIE KONDO, AUTHOR, *THE LIFE-CHANGING MAGIC OF TIDYING UP: THE JAPANESE ART OF DECLUTTERING AND ORGANIZING*

Purging the household of clutter and cleaning to accomplish a debris-free zone will give you a feeling of satisfaction, deep pleasure, gratification, and fulfillment from your achievement. Most importantly, your house is now awesome!

According to the 2017 United States Census Bureau, there are about 126 million households in the United States. That number does not include the off-the-grid yurts. Our home is where we lay our head, rest, recover, unwind, prepare food, store our chocolate ice cream, shampoo our hair, and shower up for another day in the whirlwind of life. Whether it's a glorious estate, tiny house, or studio apartment, it's where we feel safety, comfort, and at ease with ourselves, our family, and our friends. Our self-esteem and self-love need to have a safe place to land.

Making your place into a home is your safety net, your protective shell from the hectic pace of the world around you. It's where you dwell. It's where you are most yourselves. Everything in it and everything about it should be supportive to your life. Changing what's around you, changes you—how you think and feel.

## THE BUTTERFLY EFFECT

The butterfly effect is a poetic notion that the flap of a butterfly's wing in the Brazilian rain forest can cause an atmospheric effect that will spur a tornado in Oklahoma. It may take a very, very long time, but the connection is real. Collective small changes can have significant consequences around the world.

Globally, 663 million people live without access to clean drinking water, but a whopping 2.4 billion people lack access to sanitation facilities.[72] What's surprising in these statistics is the disproportion between the access to clean water and access to sanitation facilities. Water contaminated by human waste sewage can cause waterborne diseases such as cholera, typhoid, and dysentery that can have deadly effects.

One morning, an article in the *New York Times* caught billionaire Bill and Melinda Gate's attention. The headline read, "For Third World, Water Is Still a Deadly Drink." The article was about children around

163

the world dying from waterborne illnesses, in particular, diarrhea from sewage that had seeped into the water supply contaminating the drinking water.

Today, the Center for Disease Control and Prevention reports 2,195 children die every day from diarrhea. That's the equivalent of thirty-two school buses full of children needlessly dying from a largely preventable disease, diarrhea.[73]

What good is it to have access to water if it's contaminated with sewage that will make you sick? Bill and Melinda Gates felt the same and wondered why? How could it be that this is happening in the world today? This got the two of them thinking about what could be done.

The Bill & Melinda Gates Foundation is the world's largest foundation, spending nearly five billion dollars a year working on education, family planning, vaccines for the poor, and a whole host of other projects to make the world a better place, including supporting the organization WASH.[74]

WASH stands for water, sanitation, and hygiene. The primary focus of most worldwide philanthropic work is to provide clean drinking water, but little attention is on the other end—sanitation and treatment of human waste.

One in three people globally lacks sanitation, which encompasses three main things: toilets, sewer systems and sanitation facilities. The United States was built with all this in mind. Vast networks of plumbing bring clean water to just about every household. Toilets and sewage pipes take it away, off to sanitation facilities for processing. Developing third-world countries were not built with plumbing and sanitation in mind. It would be cost-prohibitive to try to bring plumbing in after the fact. It's a system that can't cost-effectively scale-down to the poorest countries.

Bill Gates decided the whole system needed to be revamped, both toilets and sanitation systems, into a new water-efficient process that would turn human waste into energy and clean by-products. Was it possible? Could a toilet not only collect waste but turn it into fuel, creating enough energy to run itself? Would it be possible for a toilet to work without pipes or even outside water?[75]

Bill and Melinda decided to throw the weight of their foundation into action, launching the "Reinvent the Toilet Challenge" in 2012. With more than half the world's population using unsafe, faulty sanitation facilities or no sanitation facilities, the mission was clear: revolutionize how we deal with pee and poop.

In 2018, prototype toilets were developed and installed in disadvantaged areas, and new sewage treatment facilities were developed too. Both are focused on taking the waste and transforming it to energy or by-products free of deadly pathogens.

> **When people thrive physically, economies grow.**
> **Poverty goes down. The world gets better.**
> —BILL GATES, FOUNDER OF MICROSOFT

It will take years, but it will happen.

On planet Earth, the interconnectedness of people the world over has an effect. In a whole-world, global philosophy, the butterfly effect has become more than poetic: it's real. We're all in this together.

> **All lives have value.**
> —BILL GATES

# WE FEEL IT IN OUR BONES

Our health, well-being, safety, and security in the world depends on countless factors. We see and hear danger approaching. When weather conditions change and become dangerous, we sense it and take shelter. We can smell rotting food to avoid eating it, and we can taste sweet fruits that are at the peak of ripeness, full of nutrients. We keep the body protected from extreme climate swings through clothing and shelter. We seek out clean air, water, and food to provide the nutrients for our body's survival. Our senses are scanning the situation, protecting us from things in the world that could do us harm. That's why we always look before crossing the street.

*We live on the leash of our senses.*

—DIANE ACKERMAN, AMERICAN POET AND NATURALIST

Stressors can ignite our fight-or-flight mode. Do we stand our ground and fight, or do we flee and get the hell out of danger's way? It's more than just surviving the elements and stresses of the world. It's not about the absence of negative things—that's not going to happen. Traffic, torrential rain, loud restaurants, or someone blocking the aisle with their shopping cart are not going away. If you live in this world, you learn to navigate it, and the minefields of problems that comes with it. That's okay. Awareness will help you manage your stress and put it in perspective.

*Our senses convey that all is not*
*well with the natural world.*

—PETER GARRETT, AUSTRALIAN CONSERVATION FOUNDATION

## CHAPTER SUMMARY

☑ We're all part of this global interdependence, diversity of cultures, and sustainability. Every life has value.

☑ Take a vacation with the eyes and see nature as the eyes are the windows to the brain. Experience a sense of awe.

☑ Focus on health and well-being. Life is a one-way ticket. Make it a good ride.

☑ Actual fear is different from perceived fear. Don't stress out over things outside your control.

☑ External clutter is internal clutter on display. Organize your dwelling to show your love and authentic self.

# PART THREE

---

# Somewhere Else

*The human brain has one hundred billion neurons,
each neuron connected to ten thousand other
neurons. Sitting on your shoulders is the most
complicated object in the known universe.*
—MICHIO KAKU, THEORETICAL PHYSICIST AND FUTURIST

*The soul is your innermost being. The presence that you
are beyond form. The consciousness that you are beyond
form, that is the soul. That is who you are in essence.*
—ECKHART TOLLE, WRITER

## THE SPAN OF A UNIVERSE IN A PEA

The most complicated part of being human is to figure out what's going on in our head. It's where learning happens, memory is stored, behaviors are generated, and perception is realized. It also controls movement, speech, emotions and a whole host of other stuff. It's our consciousness, all stuffed into a three-pound wrinkly, fatty mass contained in our noggin. The brain is the most astonishing and intricate part of the human body and it's hard to believe such complicated workings can go on inside such a small space. It's like compress the span of the universe into a pea.

In the following section, Part Three: Somewhere Else, we go into the stratosphere of somewhere else, the magical place we call consciousness. We scratch the surface of the things that affect our consciousness, how we can get derailed, what drives our decisions, what motivates our behavior, sparks our curiosity, and how love or lack of it is crucial to our very existence and on. There isn't a book big enough to explain the mysteries and complexity of what we call consciousness. I only offer a few needles I found in the haystack.

CHAPTER TEN

# Consciousness

*Most folks are about as happy as they
make up their minds to be.*

—ABRAHAM LINCOLN, SIXTEENTH PRESIDENT OF THE UNITED STATES

Happiness, isn't that what our lives are all about? But where does happiness exist?

Nothing will make you happy until you choose to be happy. No person, job, or amount of money will make you happy until you decide to be happy. Your happiness will not come to you. It can only come from you. Happiness is a choice. Like all choices, it's the little doable decisions along the way that snowball into greatness.

Let's break it down.

Maslow's level one and two, Physiological Needs and Safety Needs, deal with a part of our world where we use our senses to perceive our bodies and our surroundings. We can see, hear, touch, smell, and use all our instincts and senses to keep ourselves alive and safe in our environment. It's our physical world. It's all real: our body is real, and our surroundings are real.

What's going on inside our brain is something different. We can't see our consciousness, or smell it, or feel it. We know it's created in the brain through a ball of intertwined neurons and chemicals. Our consciousness is inherent to our existence. It's not happening in the real, physical world. It's happening somewhere else, and that somewhere else is what living mindfully is about.

> *I need one of those baby monitors from my*
> *subconscious to my consciousness so I can*
> *know what the hell I'm really thinking about.*
> —STEVEN WRIGHT, COMEDIAN

## LIFE, LIBERTY, AND THE PURSUIT OF HAPPINESS

The famous phrase in the Declaration of Independence, "life, liberty, and the pursuit of happiness," is from a centuries-old document that theoretically could have been the basis for Maslow's hierarchy of needs.

> *We hold these truths to be self-evident, that all men are*
> *created equal, that they are endowed by their Creator*
> *with certain unalienable Rights, that among these are*
> *Life, Liberty, and the pursuit of Happiness.*

Life is covered by Maslow's first level—Physiology, which deals with our bodies' needs to keep us alive.

Liberty is concerned with the second level—Safety, which deals with having a safe environment, security, and the freedom to move unobstructed in society.

The pursuit of happiness is expressed in Maslow's third and fourth levels, which deal with our consciousness and everything that makes us happy.

The third level, Love and Belonging, represents our connectedness with other people and our emotions. Love is probably the most profound human emotion you can have.

The fourth level, Esteem, explains our sense of purpose. It's the motivation to our life's purpose and to pursue a satisfying future.

Exploration of Maslow's third and fourth levels will bring a clearer understanding of what's needed to set you on the road to happiness in your life. Happiness doesn't exist in the natural world. It exists in our brain, where our emotions and intellect flourish.

Biologically, happiness manifests itself in the brain as a stew of neurochemicals: endorphins, dopamine, serotonin, oxytocin, and adrenaline. The soup of neurochemicals changes with our experiences. A dash of dopamine from a child's hug. A cup of adrenaline from watching a horror movie. The brain's chemistry changes depending on our experiences. Measuring happiness is impossible as it's uniquely subjective.

> *Buddha in India and the Stoic philosophers in ancient Greece and Rome all counseled people to break their emotional attachments to people and events, which are always unpredictable and uncontrollable, and to cultivate instead an attitude of acceptance. This ancient idea deserves respect, and it is certainly true that changing your mind is usually a more effective response to frustration than is changing the world.*
> —JONATHAN HAIDT, THE HAPPINESS HYPOTHESIS

Therefore, some researchers view happiness as two things happening simultaneously: the presence of happiness-inducing stimuli, and the absence of unhappiness-making stimuli. At the root, our road to happiness begins with the absence of pain and displeasure.[76]

Sigmund Freud posited that we as human beings are always striving to be happy, or at the very least, trying to escape pain and unhappiness.

# MARSHMALLOWS AND HAPPINESS

In 1970, two Stanford University psychologists conducted a series of experiments to try and understand when delayed gratification—the ability to wait to get something one wants—developed in children.[77] The experiment was devised to see if the early development of delayed gratification was an indication of future success.

The original experiment may have had a few flaws. For example, experimenters used a small group of participants, and the participants were not a representation of the general population's, demographic or economic status. Nonetheless, the experiment itself was a fascinating concept, and has been repeated over the years.

The experiment had children, ages seven to nine, come into a room one by one. They were asked to sit patiently and wait.

The catch was there was a sweet treat sitting on a plate in front of them. The proposition was if the child could wait until the experimenter came back into the room, approximately fifteen minutes later, they would get two sweet treats. If they didn't want to wait, they could eat one treat right away, but there would be no second treat. The sweet treat varied but the rules were the same for all the children.

There are several videos on YouTube repeating the experiment but using marshmallows as the treat. What interested me was how the kids reacted to the marshmallow just sitting there. It was a showdown—them staring at the marshmallow, and the marshmallow lusciously staring back.

In the YouTube videos, the children used fascinating tactics to fend off the urge to eat the tasty morsel. Some kids tried to distract themselves by fidgeting and looking away. Others repeatedly touched the marshmallow, lifting it for closer inspection, smelling it, and pretending to eat it; there was even a lick here and there.

The brain doesn't like resistance. The intense desire for immediate gratification has to be subjugated for the longer-term reward. The children had to manage their attention and resist the temptation to let desire breakdown their control.

Those kids who gave up and ate the one marshmallow may not have developed a strong sense of self-discipline. Or for some kids, the reward of the second marshmallow wasn't worth the wait. The experiment may have fallen short of proving that early development of delayed gratification correlates to future success. That's a big assumption to make from a marshmallow—and as adults, the stakes are much higher. Now, we're talking about a whole lot more than just marshmallows.

As adults, we continually face situations that can cause us discomfort or pain. We want everything now. Doing it now gives pleasure now. Now is now, now is much better than later. As a result, we often give in to the immediate pleasure, the instant gratification to avoid the pain of resistance.

### *Instant gratification takes too long.*
#### —CARRIE FISHER, AUTHOR, *POSTCARDS FROM THE EDGE*

There're are two types of pleasure, both of which affect our ability to resist instant gratification.

First, there are instinctual, or physical pleasures.

We have a complicated relationship with pleasure as it's also related to our instincts and survival. Satisfying the primal instincts of hunger, thirst, and sex is also pleasurable. Sex gives us a thrill as well as protects the survival of the species. Satisfying these primal instincts feels good. For God's sake, we want to eat the marshmallow already! Intense cravings and instinctual drives muddy our ability to think clearly and reason.

We can find an early example of this internal conflict in the poem *Metamorphoses* by Ovid. In the poem, Eros, the primordial god of love and sex, shoots Medea with his arrow. Medea is struck, and says, "I am dragged along by a strange new force. Desire and reason are pulling in different directions. I see the right way and approve it, but follow the wrong."

There are also psychological pleasures.

One example of this type of pleasure is vanity. Vanity is excessive admiration of one's appearance. Many of us are tempted to look our best, even at a high cost. Do we splurge on the latest designer outfit or save the money for our financial future—so far away? Both choices offer a certain psychological satisfaction or pleasure. The immediate gratification and thrill of a new outfit or to have the future happiness of financial security. It's the choice between a more immediate reward or a future reward. Developing a tolerance for waiting may even give higher value to the future life goals.

> *We've all been raised on television to believe that one day we'd all be millionaires, and movie gods, and rock stars. But we won't. And we're slowly learning that fact. And we're very, very pissed off.*
> —TYLER DURDEN, NARRATOR OF THE MOVIE *FIGHT CLUB*

We sometimes confuse pleasure with happiness. Pleasures are short-lived experiences. The thrill of having the new outfit fades. The happiness that comes from having financial security is long term. An extreme of self-indulgent pleasure could spark an addiction, whether to substances or behaviors. With happiness, there's no such thing as getting too much.

# THE ELEPHANT AND THE RIDER

Johnathan Haidt, professor of ethical leadership at New York University, uses the analogy of a rider and elephant to explain how the two independent systems in the brain can work together or be in conflict. There's the rational or intellectual system of the brain that's represented by the rider. The emotional system is represented by the elephant.

The rider sits up high on top of the elephant, sees the path ahead, makes the decisions and guides the elephant. The rider appears to be in charge, but if there's a disagreement between the rider and the elephant, the elephant, being much larger, could easily resist and do what it wants.

The elephant, or our emotional system, provides the power to take the journey and attain our goals. But the elephant, like our emotional system, prefers quick gratification and doesn't usually look that far ahead to long-term rewards. The elephant can be directed by the rider, but the elephant could just as easily do nothing, dump the rider off, go play with other elephants, or head off to the nearest mango tree for a snack.

It's that power imbalance that makes adapting new habits, lifestyle changes, and behaviors hard. The trick is the elephant and rider need to move together for progress to take place.

In order for this to happen, think about the journey or path ahead. It needs to be obstacle-free, as short as possible, and the rider has to have clear direction on the plan to get to the destination. The rider also has to emotionally engage the elephant so the elephant is happy to go on the journey. All these things add to the progress, shape the path ahead, and aid in attaining your goals.

The rider, or our rational brain, is responsible for making plans, knowing the direction and motivating the elephant to do what's needed. The rider does the planning but sometimes can gets overwhelmed or exhausted with deciphering the choices. This is when the elephant sees its opportunity to willy-nilly do what it pleases.[78]

We've all experienced this emotional versus rational conflict. For instance, you decide you want to improve your level of fitness and put together a workout schedule. Your *rider* plans to hit the gym at 6:00 a.m. before work four days a week. One day a few weeks later, you're overwhelmed with a project at work. Instead of going to bed on time you relax by binge watching a new TV series. The next morning you oversleep and miss your workout session. Missing the workouts becomes more and more frequent until you abandon the early morning training sessions altogether. The *rider* was exhausted and too distracted to direct the *elephant* to get adequate sleep and make it to the gym on time.

This is why adopting new behaviors can be challenging. To keep our elephant on course and motivated, we need to remove obstacles and make the elephant's journey purposeful. A bored elephant tends to wander, and since elephants live in herds, they tend to do whatever all the other elephants are doing.

## THE TWO SIDES OF DECISIONS—INTELLECT AND EMOTIONS

What raises humans above all other animals is our ability to reason and our unbounded emotional drive. *Homo sapiens* have the highest intellect and are the most emotional animals on Earth.

Our decisions define us, but it's the decision-making process that may seem like a negotiation between our intellectual reasoning and our emotional feelings. Reasoning requires us to transcend our other emotions, our desires, our impulses, and our instincts. But it's our emotions that give us passions, intuition, creativity, and enthusiasm.

Intellect without emotion leaves no room for compassion or empathy. Everything is viewed as rational, even robotic.

Emotion without intelligence leaves no room for pragmatic goals, systematic achievements, logic, or structure.

It's complicated.

Think of the mind split into two halves of a pendulum's swinging arc.

One side processes intellectual thought: 2 + 2 = 4. There's not much emotional content in an equation. At best, you hope you were smart enough to get it right.

The other arc depicts the emotional side of the mind, motivated to make decisions based on compassion, desires, instincts, passion, and love. Sometimes decisions made by the emotional brain make no intellectual sense at all, but we're driven to make them anyway. For example, when Eros shot Medea with the arrow of desire.

As the pendulum swings back and forth, you can address any decision with pure intellect, or with pure emotions. Most often, we look at both sides of the coin or both sides of the arc and make our decision with a blend of rationality and emotion.

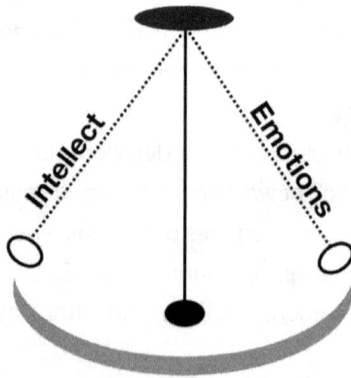

**DECISION-MAKING PROCESS
BETWEEN INTELLECT AND EMOTIONS**

## "LITTLE BOY" AND "FAT MAN"

In 1945, the United States, with the support of its allies the United Kingdom and the Republic of China, dropped two nuclear bombs on two cities
in Japan, Hiroshima and Nagasaki. The bomb named "Little Boy" was
dropped on Hiroshima on August 6, and the bomb "Fat Man," over Nagasaki
on August 9. To date, these are the only two nuclear bombs used in a war.

Nazi Germany had surrendered a few months earlier on May 8, 1945,
ending the war in Europe, but Japan was still at war with the world. The
United States and its allies felt there was no choice: it was imperative to
bring swift closure to a war that could have been very long and costly
in terms of both dollars and human lives.

To prepare, the United States initially called for an unconditional surrender of the Japanese in the Potsdam Declaration of July 26th, 1945, and
threatened Japan with "prompt and utter destruction." Japan ignored
the ultimatum, and within a few days, the bombs were deployed.

The long-term effects of the bombs were linked to approximately 90,000
to 166,000 deaths of the people of Hiroshima and 60,000 to 80,000
deaths of the people living in Nagasaki. About half the deaths occurred
in the first few days after the bombs were dropped.

On August 15, 1945, six days after the last bomb was dropped, Japan
announced its surrender. The ethical justification for the bombing of
Japan is and probably always will be debated, despite the intellectual
reasoning behind the decision.

## LET THE PENDULUM SWING—INTELLECTUAL CHOICE

On an intellectual basis, correlations were made between the future cost
of bombing Japan and not bombing Japan—in dollars, effectiveness, and

human lives—while the strengths and abilities of the Japanese Army compared to our own were carefully assessed.

The Imperial Japanese Army, rooted in samurai tradition with exceptional loyalty to the emperor of Japan, had amassed approximately 5.5 million men by 1945, the height of World War II. They were famed for their kamikaze pilots. *Kamikaze,* which means "God's wind," were a special unit task force that was sent on one-way, bombing attacks, and nearly four thousand kamikaze pilots were sacrificed to these suicide missions.

The Japanese military was equipped and prepared for a long fight. The attack on the United States Navy at Pearl Harbor on December 7, 1941, is "a date which will live in infamy." That's how President Franklin D. Roosevelt described the situation and as the day the United States was pulled into World War II.

In terms of equipment, ships, and military personnel, the attack inflicted enormous devastation on the United States. The naval fleet at Pearl Harbor was decimated, with nine ships sunk and twenty-one ships badly damaged. The death toll of 2,402 was mostly military personnel.

Within an hour of the speech by President Roosevelt, Congress passed a formal declaration of war against Japan that officially brought the United States into World War II.

Over four years later, the devastation of the American fleet at Pearl Harbor was still on the mind of President Harry S. Truman when he made the decision to bomb Japan. In the hearts and minds of most Americans, it was the hardest decision ever made. President Harry S. Truman wrote, "Nobody is more disturbed over the use of Atomic bombs than I am, but I was greatly disturbed over the unwarranted attack by the Japanese on Pearl Harbor and their murder of our prisoners of war. The only language they seem to understand is the one we have been using to bombard them."

The intellectual reasoning to use the bomb relied heavily on the assumption that not using it would cost the United States at least an additional five hundred thousand American lives to bring the war to an end.

The decision was made to drop the bombs on Hiroshima and Nagasaki because of the two cities' military and industrial significance, and in doing so could cost the Japanese approximately two hundred thousand lives. In the end, the calculation to save five hundred thousand American lives outweighed the cost of two hundred thousand Japanese lives.

The final nail in the coffin was the hypothesis that dropping the bombs would stop Japan and would also bring an end to World War II. During the six years of World War II, world-wide some seventy-five million people had died. Accurate numbers were never ascertained, but it's believed world-wide about twenty million were military personnel and about forty million were civilians. To President Harry Truman, and those involved with making the decision, two hundred thousand Japanese lives may have seemed a small price pay to avoid any further loss of American lives and to bring an end to the war. Most important, ending the war would end the killing and allow the world to then move on and heal.

> ### *I'm against sloppy, emotional thinking.*
> —HERMAN KAHN, MILITARY STRATEGIST, ANALYZING THE LIKELY
> CONSEQUENCES OF NUCLEAR WAR

## LET THE PENDULUM SWING—EMOTIONAL CHOICE

On a purely emotional basis, we're talking about human life here, and therefore the emotional toll of lost lives, lost love, and a lost generation. Is there any justification for the decimation of human life? The true answer lies in your moral compass and where along the arc of the pendulum swing would you find grounds to cast your vote to use or not use the bomb. What justification would you use, if any?

**_Eye for an eye, tooth for a tooth._**
—EXODUS 21:24

The eye for an eye principle was founded in Babylonian law around 1780 BC. Also, the Jewish Talmud interprets the verses referring to "an eye for an eye" to mean reasonable compensation for monetary damages, and that a person who has injured another person is penalized to a similar degree. Again, this is intellectually consistent and may seem fair if you're talking about monetary compensation to fix one's car after an accident, but what about human life? If you're rooted in the emotional arc of the pendulum's apex, then the act of taking a life for a life ups the ante to a morally uncomfortable and unconscionable level. Is a life for a life considered fair and reasonable compensation?

**_An eye for an eye makes the whole world blind._**
—MAHATMA GANDHI

Mahatma Gandhi was the preeminent leader of Indian nationalism against British-ruled India. He advocated a course of nonviolence during his life and even took on a vegetarian lifestyle that represented his nonviolence against animals. Although the policy of nonviolence was famously used during Gandhi's campaign for independence in India, Gandhi may have never actually said the now-famous quote above, which was attributed to him by the biographer Louis Fischer. Whatever the case, Mr. Gandhi was successful, and in 1947 the British government agreed to withdraw from India, and India became an independent and sovereign nation.

**_Our emotional symptoms are precious_**
**_sources of life and individuality._**
—SAINT THOMAS MORE, PHILOSOPHER AND STATESMAN

Rooted in our conscious is how we decides to approach a decision. The swinging of the pendulum between the two apexes of intelligent choice and emotional choice leaves a whole lot of a gray area in between. It's the struggle between the two aspects of our mind that makes us human. It gives us angst, feelings, reasoning, integrity, and courage, and it drives every decision we make, from the mundane choice of what color to paint our kitchen to whether we should press the button that drops the next nuclear bomb. It's the essence of why we exist, and of why we're human.

# THE TWO SIDES—INTELLECT AND EMOTIONS

We possess such superior intellects that the technologies we've created (e.g., the very fact you're able to read this page), our self-expression through the arts and the development of family social structures, kinships, social norms, moral values, and philosophies—even putting a man on the moon—leave any other form of life on earth in the proverbial atmospheric dust.

We are the rock stars in the genetic, evolutionary timeline. All because we possess two more important qualities than our fellow planetary species: we have the greatest intellectual and emotional capacity of all. We're driven to excel, to be the best in our class, to find meaningful relationships, to have fulfilling careers, and to create spiritual connections with others, our God, and our faiths, whatever they may be.

Our intellectual and emotional capacity is wrapped up in one very intricate part of our being human: our brain, mind, or consciousness. The mind is the split personality, a two-part system that can waiver between making intellectual choices rooted in systematic logic or passionate decisions rooted in emotions.

How our mind makes decisions, through our thoughts and emotions, is what ultimately defines our choices and defines us as individuals. Our emotional thoughts and intellectual thoughts, the two furthest points of the same swinging pendulum, are equally important and fulfilling aspects that complete us as humans. We make choices based on how we feel or what we think, and those choices, in every aspect of our lives, become us and define us.

> *There is zero correlation between IQ and*
> *emotional empathy ... They're controlled*
> *by a different part of the brain.*
> —DANIEL GOLEMAN, AUTHOR OF EMOTIONAL INTELLIGENCE

## COSMIC CONSCIOUSNESS

Our mind, our consciousness, is the most critical aspect of being human. But there's more to our consciousness outside the decision-making process. Our decisions may define us, but our consciousness is undefinable and limitless. It's our awareness.

*Merriam-Webster* defines consciousness as "the quality or state of being aware especially of something within oneself."

> *The prevailing consensus in neuroscience is that*
> *consciousness is an emergent property of the brain*
> *and its metabolism. When the brain dies, the mind*
> *and consciousness of the being to whom that brain*
> *belonged ceases to exist. In other words, without*
> *a brain there can be no consciousness.*[79]
> — CLIFFORD N. LAZARUS PH D

Our consciousness manifests in different ways. We're aware of ourselves and our surroundings when we're awake, but have an altered form of awareness when dreaming. We set ourselves apart from all other animals on the planet as having a higher form of consciousness, a cosmic consciousness, an infinite intelligence connected with the universe. It's more of an intuitive knowing than using our faculties to discern our sense of place or being. This sense of consciousness is almost void of any organic explanation, but we somehow know there's a realm greater than ourselves. This is sometimes referred to as the *God spot*.

In 1901, Richard M. Bucke published *Cosmic Consciousness: A Study in the Evolution of the Human Mind*. Bucke identified that joyfulness; a revelation of the meaning, purpose, and aliveness of the universe; a sense of immortality; a loss of fear of death; and an absence of the concept of sin as components of our expansive state of being.

For me, consciousness means to create and be a part of a beautiful world. What better place to start than with our own happiness.

## CHAPTER SUMMARY

☑ Practice gratitude. Feelings of thankfulness correlate to waiting for long-term rewards. Gratitude today can give you a stronger sense of purpose in attaining your future goals.

☑ Take time to be in the moment, appreciate the day and reconnect with your surroundings. Take a mental break to let the brain wander and day dream. Science now proves it's useful to let yourself unplug. To gain self-control, let go of self-centeredness.

☑ Accept what's outside your control and take responsibility for what is within your control.

☑ Remember, you are stronger than your self-indulgent desires.

## CHAPTER ELEVEN

# Love and Belonging

*Life is hard. Life is beautiful.*
*Life is difficult. Life is wonderful.*
—KATE DI CAMILLO, AUTHOR OF CHILDREN'S FICTION

Life is difficult, but we don't have to do it alone. That's what makes life truly joyful. We have family, friends, co-hearts, and sometimes a special someone we want to share it all with.

Our sense of belonging and love is the key to understanding the value of our life. Through shared experiences, we connect. There's a great sense of satisfaction and personal joy in any accomplishment, but the real cherry on top is our need to share it.

Love what you do, and love who you do it with.

The African proverb, "It takes a village to raise a child," means children grow through the love and interactions of the entire village, through the community. We don't get anywhere alone.

*I surround myself with good people who make*
*me feel great and give me positive energy.*
—ALI KRIEGER, FIFA WOMEN'S WORLD CUP CHAMPION

It's in our emotional space or that part of the consciousness where our spirit, soul, and heart all reside. Where we can go from tears of joy to feeling ripped apart with anger. From a state of contentment to feelings of drudgery as we make our way through the day. It's our feelings of love and connectedness with ourselves and with others that bring us joy and contentment.

It's in our emotional space where we build a network of people we hold dear. When someone close to us passes from this life it can feel as though our universe has cracked. Or having a newborn cradled in our arms can bring us overwhelming feelings of joy and deep love.

No aspect of our life is more important to the quality and meaning of our existence than our emotions with ourselves, with people in our lives, and with our spiritual beings. They're what make life worth living; unfortunately, our emotions can also lead to the depths of despair that drive some to end their existence. Emotions are responsible for our love-hate relationship with all people, and they all starts with how you love yourself.

## SELF-LOVE IS LIKE PUTTING YOUR OWN OXYGEN MASK ON FIRST

Years ago on a Valentine's Day, I was very single and had no plans for the evening. I left work around 8:00 p.m., later than usual. No big reason to rush home. The grocery store would be empty—the perfect time for shopping—and I knew the fridge was a wasteland of postmortem takeout boxes. I was surveying the roasted chickens for the crispiest exterior when a voice boomed over the intercom, "For those last-minute Valentine's Day shoppers, a dozen roses are half-priced." I thought, Okay, I'll bite. Chicken in one hand and the other arm full of roses, I headed home.

My life was pretty much in order: excellent career on track, in reasonable health with weight at 130, still young enough, owned a house and a car. I had enough money in the bank to never work again provided I was mindful and not willy-nilly about spending money.

Everything was clicking—except for the man thing. It had been a challenging year—okay, a decade of not-likely-to-go-anywhere relationships with a few hell-no dates blended in. I had concluded that maybe God meant for me to be alone in this lifetime, and I was okay with that. It was precisely a week later when I met the man I would marry—but that's a story for another time.

Now, I want to go back to me and stick with me. That's my point: it all starts with the self. Self-love. Buy yourself the roses.

"You, yourself, as much as anybody in the entire universe, deserves your love and affection." This quote is often attributed to Buddha but there's no evidence to support that fact. Regardless of who said it, it's so true. You deserve your own love.

Buddha did say, "You find no one dearer than yourself ... So you shouldn't hurt others if you love yourself." Again, love starts with you.

Let's start. What do I mean by self-love, and why should you care?

Here's a little story to illustrate my point. A male friend, let's call him Bob, had gone through a bad breakup and was ready to move onward and upward, setting out to look for his future wife. He had snagged a couple of coffee dates with a potential love interest. He was geared up for his big move, a Saturday night dinner date—pick up, drop off, and hopefully breakfast the next morning. Bob was psyched.

Thinking he might want to up his game, I asked if he would like to borrow my car for the big night. You see Bob drove a rusted-out, uphol-stery-peeling death trap that made any discussion of year, make, or model irrelevant. Bob did well and could easily afford whatever car he wanted. To Bob, his four-wheeled carcass was a statement against something I have long forgotten.

Bob was indignant at my suggestion, claiming he would never be interested in any woman who like him based on the car he drove.

This was when I had to explain self-love in man terms. "Bob, the car you drive shows how you care about yourself, and how you care about yourself is how you'll care about others—like a future wife."

A few days later, Bob bought a new, high-safety-rated Jeep Cherokee.

> *Self-care is never a selfish act— it is simply*
> *good stewardship of the only gift I have, the*
> *gift I was put on earth to offer to others.*
> —PARKER PALMER, AUTHOR OF LET YOUR LIFE SPEAK

Flash bulletin: You have control over what's on the recorded messages playing in your brain, and you can change the messages anytime you want.

Self-love is not about a new car. You can't buy self-love. It may manifest itself as a tidy lifestyle as people full of self-love tend to take better care of themselves, but it has to start on the inside with your thoughts. It's the inner voice, the ping-ponging chunks of commentary we habitually banter roll around the brain on a daily basis. The messages you've been feeding yourself, positive and negative, eventually become your firmly held beliefs.

You might think this would be an excellent time to introduce the use of positive affirmation in the whole habit-forming scenario of self-love—but not so fast. A Post-it note with YOU'RE AWESOME written on it stuck to the bathroom mirror will soon lose its stickum and fall off, only to be found when you clean behind the toilet. Just telling yourself "you're awesome" doesn't work. You need to believe it—totally, profoundly, and in your soul.

You need proof you're awesome.

Let's look at the book of Genesis. It doesn't matter whether you're religious or not; the story in Genesis is an excellent place to discover how deep your self-love must be. Genesis starts with verse 1, "In the beginning God created the heavens and earth," and over the next twenty-plus verses God creates light, darkness, waters, air, land, plants bearing seeds, trees bearing fruits, birds, creatures, livestock, and wild animals.

Then, in verse 27 he creates mankind.

> **So God created mankind in his own image, in the image of God, he created them; male and female, he created them.**
> —GENESIS 1:27

Here lies the proof that you're awesome, and that above all else you must understand this one thing. You're made out of the same divine cosmic goo as all the stars, planets, flowers, sun, moon, elephants, whales, birds, poets, painters, scientists—everyone and everything in the universe. Everything comes from the same divine energy source, whatever that may be, and whatever that may mean to you. We're all made from the same gorgeous, divine, atomic energy. Know you are truly magnificent just the way you are.

> **You are a divine creation—a being of light who showed up here as a human being at the exact moment you were supposed to ... You are the beloved, a miracle, a part of the eternal perfection.**
> —WAYNE DYER, 10 SECRETS OF SUCCESS AND INNER PEACE

Treat yourself like you would a close friend, with affection, kindness, understanding, empathy, and the occasional dash of humor. Self-love is a life skill, and it's the one gift you can give yourself every day in perpetuity. Self-love leads to self-esteem, self-confidence, and self-acceptance. Self-love is a habit, and habits need to be practiced. Essentially, self-love is the product of forming habits that support a loving relationship with yourself.

*To fall in love with yourself is the first secret to happiness.*
—ROBERT MORLEY, ENGLISH ACTOR

## ONESOME INTO A TWOSOME

If love begins with the self, then once that's on our radar, how about a special someone to share it all with?

In 2018 there were over sixty-one million married couples, representing over 55 percent of Americans age eighteen and over. Having a special someone in our life seems to be a priority for the majority—but what are the deal-breaker questions we might ask ourselves to know if this person is the one or the one to avoid? What's important in a long-term, marriage-oriented or partner-committed relationship?

## TWO QUESTIONS TO ASK YOURSELF BEFORE YOU SAY, "I DO"

As they say, love conquers all.

To be loved is one of the most fundamental human desires. Love cancels out fear, loathing, anger, and other negative emotions. To be loved and truly, deeply love someone in return creates a unique human bond.

*If you would be loved, love, and be loveable.*
—BENJAMIN FRANKLIN

Recorded evidence from 2350 BC shows ceremonies between a man and a woman. The custom of marriage was embraced by ancient civilizations and made its way through the ages to today. We've tweaked it a bit with same sex marriages but the concept of committed love is the same for all.

Divorce has also made it through the ages. Today, approximately 45 percent of first marriages end in divorce, making the odds about even that you may or may not be spending the rest of your lives together.

What should you be asking before you say, "I do"?

When I Googled "what makes a good marriage," I got lists of things you could do to make your marriage fulfilling, happy and harmonious. Like having excellent communication, a sense of humor, shared interests, showing appreciation, being trustworthy, honest, and affectionate, having sex—the advice seems endless on things to do once the wedding is over. All great suggestions, but before you tie your life to another's, there are two questions you need to ask yourself about this person.

Number one: Are they committed?
Number two: Do they make good decisions?

The first question: Are they committed?

This may seem obvious, but if you look at the original wedding vows, commitment is expressed in the most profound sense of an unbreakable life contract ... for better, for worse, for richer, for poorer, in sickness and in health, to love and to cherish, till death do us part. Love is an unconditional commitment to an imperfect person.

> *Your life changes the moment you make a new,*
> *congruent, and committed decision.*
> —TONY ROBBINS, LIFE COACH

You have to ask yourself, will this person be there for the family and me—no matter what? Are they committed physically, spiritually, emotionally, intellectually, and financially? Are they going to care years from now? Will they put me, our relationship, and the family we build before anything else, even before their ambitions and desires? Are their decisions for the good of the family, or for the good of themselves alone?"

> **We both know that no matter what, we'll be**
> **with each other—and we'll get through it.**
> —RITA WILSON, ON HER LASTING THIRTY-ONE-YEAR MARRIAGE TO
> MOVIE STAR TOM HANKS

The society we live in even recognizes this unique bond between spouses. In a court of law, marriage is regarded as a blessed union between people. Therefore, a spouse can claim *spousal privilege*. This means a spouse cannot be compelled to testify against the other spouse. Those things spouses share in confidence cannot be brought into court, compelling one spouse to rat out the other.

Also called *spousal immunity*, the court recognizes the bond of spouses, their commitment to each other and the court's obligation to protect and promote marital felicity. What's said in private between spouses is protected by marital privilege. In 1839, the Supreme Court called marriage "the best solace of human existence."

> **Unless commitment is made, there are only**
> **promises and hopes; but no plans.**
> —PETER F. DRUCKER, CELEBRATED AS THE MAN WHO INVENTED MANAGEMENT

So, ask yourself:

Is this person committed?
Are they in 100 percent?
Are they committed to the relationship, to your future family and you?

Now let's explore question number two: Do they make good decisions?

Life is made up of an infinite number of choices. What you eat, where you live, what line of work to pursue; some big decisions, some small, but still, decisions to be made.

> ***Life is about choices. Some we regret, some we're proud of. Some will haunt us forever. The message: we are what we choose to be.***
> —GRAHAM BROWN, AMERICAN WRITER

Also, equally important is how a person makes decisions.

Do they confront the options with courage, or procrastinate, afraid of making the wrong decision?

Do they revel in the chance to create the life they want to live, or succumb to the mediocrity of indecisiveness?

You can't make progress without making decisions. The person you are about to tether your life to needs to be making good ones—better yet, outstanding ones.

Making good decisions is not easy. You're not one decision but a collection of years of decisions, which shape your life along with your partner's life.

Life is like walking on the edge of a knife: you could easily fall to either side. It takes strength and balance to stay on the straight and narrow of the blade. Sometimes you get pushed off the edge by others and therein lies the choice. Who you surround yourself with, especially when it comes to a spouse or partner, makes it easier to maintain your balance and strength—if they're making great decisions too.

*The key to accepting responsibility for your life is to accept the fact that your choices, every one of them, are leading you inexorably to either success or failure, however you define those terms.*
—NEAL BOORTZ, TALK RADIO HOST

Mistakes will be made along the way. We're human and subject to error. But there's a vast difference between making mistakes and making bad decisions. Selecting the wrong answer on a test is a mistake; not studying for that test is a bad decision. Mistakes are things that happen without intention. Bad decisions, however negligent or intentional they may be, are made without thinking ahead toward the consequences. Bad decisions have bad outcomes.

We negotiate our bad decisions and sometimes try to reclassify them as mistakes, but this only fools the fool. Falling into a rut, not evaluating future consequences, not thinking it through are all part of the process of making a bad decision. Bad decisions that have become habits may have adverse effects on the progress of your life, and your partner's life too.

You make the decisions day after day to eat high-caloric, fatty, and sugary foods that cause you to gain weight over time. This lifestyle habit may eventually affect your overall health. Obesity is the leading cause of heart disease and diabetes. The long-term consequences of what you eat today may not be on your mind when you're chowing down on fried foods, but it should be. It's the smallness of your decisions that, in the future, may be the ones that affect you most. It's not what you have for lunch today but what you decide to have for lunch every day.

People who are broken—who continue to make extremely bad decisions that are a detriment to their future—may very well be addicts of some nature. They're not functional, responsible adults. You can't fix them. You can love them, but trying to fix them will potentially do more harm than good. Broken people have to fix their own life first before they can be there for someone else.

For example, the person you're seeing may be caught up in drugs, alcohol, or a whole plethora of unhealthy, bad habits. An alcoholic is incapable of making a committed decision. Their first commitment is not even to themselves but to the alcohol. They may love you and say they're committed, but that person is not truly themselves. Even the courts recognize an intoxicated person cannot legally enter into a contract, thereby making the contract voidable. First and foremost, they're tied to their addiction, whether it's drugs or alcohol, gambling, hoarding, overspending or other unwanted behaviors.

Many people suffering from depression or other mental disorders may self-medicate with drugs, alcohol, gambling, sex or other behaviors. We can only love and support them. They have to be the one, with their own courage, to change themselves.

But even the worst alcoholic or drug addict, through their hard work, can change and transcend their old bad decisions, habits, and lifestyle. It's a journey they need to make alone. They're not available for a commitment and are in the beginning stage of forming a string of new good decisions to lead them to a better life. People with a history of alcohol or drug abuse who have transcended their disease are some of the strongest people I know. It takes an enormous amount of time, courage, and work to get sober, stay sober, and build a new life of sobriety.

> *You can't go back and make a new start, but you can start right now and make a brand new ending.*
> —JAMES R. SHERMAN, AMERICAN WRITER

On the other hand, good decisions positively impact yourself and others. Having a healthy lifestyle will result in being there for yourself and being able to do the physical things you want. You'll be there for your spouse, your kids, your friends and the world.

Dating is the time to get to know a person. Figure out what makes them tick, see if they're true to themselves, if they're a good person, and if their weirdness complements your weirdness. If your ultimate goal is marriage, or to have a life partner, then somewhere in the process you're going to be taking a hard look at this person. Ask yourself the two most important questions: Are they committed, and do they make good decisions?

As you're figuring it out, get out a mirror, take a good look at yourself. Ask the same two questions about yourself. Rest assured, your potential spouse or life partner is asking themselves the very same questions about you.

And by the way, get your own crap in order. Your past will come back to haunt you too. Spend the time now to become the person you would want to date or marry. Get it together, because no one is going to fix you—only you can fix you.

> *People are sent into our lives to teach us things*
> *that we need to learn about ourselves.*
> —MANDY HALE, AUTHOR

## PEOPLE WHO NEED PEOPLE

People we love are all the people who touch our life, from the person we choose as our spouse or life partner to the person who says hello while passing us on the street. It's all degrees of love, from a smidgen of kindness to an outright, open-hearted, full-on love fest. We seek love and belonging, from large social groups to the person we want to spend our life with. We need love in our lives.

*I cannot even imagine where I would be today were it not*
*for that handful of friends who have given me a heart full*
*of joy. Let's face it, friends make life a lot more fun.*

−CHARLES R. SWINDOLL, CHRISTIAN PASTOR

Picture a good-sized dot with concentric rings expanding outward around it. You're the dot. You're the center of your universe.

Then all the people in your life are placed somewhere on one of the expanding concentric circles. Some are on closer circles, and some are on the outer rings. On the outermost ring might be the homeless man who asked you for spare change. A little closer might be the barista at the coffee shop who knows you like almond milk in your latte.

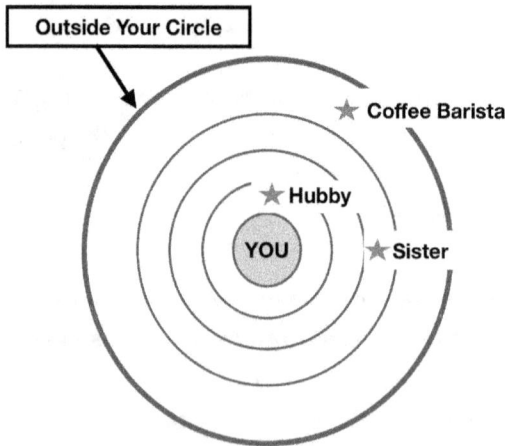

CIRCLE OF PEOPLE IN YOUR LIFE

These are all people who, even on the periphery of your life, have an impact. A thank-you wave from the guy you let merge into your lane of traffic can take your morning commute from unbearable to a sing-along with the radio. It's these little speed bumps of love hits that can affect your overall feeling of well-being throughout the day.

The Golden Rule is found in Luke 6:31, which records Jesus to have said, "Do to others as you would have them do to you." The second commandment of the Bible is, "Love your neighbor as yourself." This all sums up a world of harmonic utopia where everyone is looking out for each other no matter where they fall on those concentric expanding rings.

Relationships change. People may move closer or farther out on the rings depending on your relationship with them. When your house is under construction, your architect may be on a circle just past your spouse. Once the house has the official certificate of occupancy from the city permit department, your architect may drift to a status on a ring similar to those living in the hinterlands of the Siberian peninsula. We ebb and flow with the closeness or usefulness of people in our lives by shared needs, companionship, partnerships, workplace hierarchy, team sports, and common goals.

We need people. We need their love, support, friendship, and cowork, and they need us—but it may not always be a perfect match.

## LIFE-CHALLENGING EVENT NUMBER THREE—BUT IT'S NOT MY LIFE THIS TIME

My brother had been diagnosed with polycystic kidney disease, a degenerative disease that causes the kidneys to form polyps. Over time, the kidneys lose their ability to function and eventually fail. My brother's kidneys were fading with less than 10 percent function, and the doctors wanted to do an immediate transplant before they failed completely.

This is when the hospital transplant coordinator would contact all willing family members to see if they would donate a kidney. Then a genetic test is performed to determine whether any family members are a tissue match. My two other brothers that were ready, willing, and, hopefully, able to be donors. They were going to do the test, and I thought—Hooray—they have it covered.

I was recently engaged, and my head was swimming with wedding plans, floral arrangements, and guest lists as the wedding was less than two months away. After a preliminary conversation with the hospital transplant coordinator, she swayed me to throw my genetic hat into the ring as well. She kept saying I was probably not a match. She explained I was much smaller than my brother and probably not a match. I was a girl and probably not a match. With every question she asked she ended with saying I was probably not going to be a match. Not to be concerned, she explained, most family members are not a match, but as a hard rule, they test all eligible family members at the same time. Off to the doctor for a blood draw—I didn't think much about it since I was "probably not a match," or so she predicted.

I was driving along, my engagement ring casting a disco ball sparkle over the cockpit of my car. It made me think of fireflies. I was listening to an oldies radio station, and the Dixie Cups' 1964 rendition of "(Going to the) Chapel of Love" just happened to provide the background music to my disco-ball flickers. "Going to the chapel and we're gonna get married. Going to the chapel of love." The tunes were cranking, fireflies flittering, and I was in a pre-bridal euphoria—until the phone rang. I recognized the number. It was the hospital transplant coordinator.

She had good news! Wonderful. One of my siblings was a match, and all would be well. I asked which brother. She explained it wasn't one of my brothers—it was me. Not only was I a match, I was a 100 percent genetic match, which was apparently extremely rare.

Stunned, I briefly time-lapsed back to academia recalling that I had never, in my life, gotten a hundred percent score on a test, and why now? But this was not that kind of test.

We talked briefly about follow-up. I would need an angiogram of the arterial structure of my kidneys. She expressed the urgency of the operation. Finally, I said I needed to talk to my fiancé before I could even think about anything else. After all, it was only a few weeks until our wedding, and a lot of balls were in motion.

I made my way home and relayed the late-breaking news to my fiancé. I remember babbling, trying to convince myself this was all doable. Like scheduling a hair appointment, I could slip into the hospital right after the wedding and donate an organ, or maybe I could squeeze it in between dress fittings before the wedding.

My fiancé sat patiently, waiting for my emotions to catch up to reality. He paused, (he's an excellent decision maker) then announced we needed to cancel the wedding so I could be emotionally free to do what I needed to do. I knew he was right, but I broke into tears anyway. I had him make all the calls to cancel everything. I couldn't do it.

A few weeks later, I went under anesthesia, and they took my left kidney and gingerly placed it into the pelvic cavity of my brother. It immediately started to produce urine. My brother would be okay. It amazes me that you can take a whole organ from a living person and put it in another person. It's a miracle.

Some scientists attest organs have a cellular memory, and an organ recipient may take on the personality traits of the donor. But no, my brother did not start wearing cuter outfits or have the desire to start attending ladies' tea parties. Nothing much changed about him.

*Anger is an acid that can do more harm to the vessel in which it is stored than to anything on which it is poured.*

—MARK TWAIN.

The inconsistencies in my brother's nature were always something I had a hard time dealing with. Like being on a trampoline, sometimes he's up, sometimes he's down. He could be funny—downright hilarious—and then turn angry, ripping into you—sometimes in unbearable ways. With him, I felt it was always a pins-and-needles situation to see if you were going to get the hilarious brother or the other one.

The Buddha compared holding on to anger to grasping a hot coal with the intent of throwing it at someone else. You, of course, are the one who gets burned.

In the following months, friends learned of my donation. They expressed mixed opinions on whether they would have done the same for their brother. Over the years, it became apparent my brother and I couldn't form a relationship that nurtured either of us and we eventually just stop talking to each other. I do miss the hilarious brother though.

**_Silence is one of the hardest arguments to refute._**
—JOSH BILLINGS, AMERICAN HUMORIST

I willingly gave him my left kidney, but not because we were close or ever hoped to become close. Although at times, I naïvely thought maybe we could. We just didn't resonate. There wasn't any harmony between us. The kidney donation wasn't about the two of us—it was about the circle of people that revolved around both our lives. It was the fact that he was my mother's son, my sister-in-law's husband, and my niece's father. The value of his life was bigger than the two of us. It affected so many of those we both loved.

A friend explained to me that in the Jewish faith, this would be a _mitzvah_, or the best of selfless deeds, and I would be assured a place in heaven. The same accolade came from a Christian friend who said this type of sacrifice is of the highest order, and I was an angel. It was my Buddhist friend who put things in perspective. The Buddhists and Hindus believe in karma—a person's actions in previous lives affect their existing life. She wondered, what egregious infraction I could have done to my brother in an earlier life that I owed him a kidney in this one?

That karma rocked my perspective.

Many people said I was a hero, but it was misplaced praise. Although the donation process does involve a great deal of pain for the donor, a month later, I was driving myself to the salon for a much-needed manicure and pedicure spa appointment, and I've had no major health problems from the donation. The true heroes are those people waiting and waiting for the possible life-changing, life-saving organ transplant. To keep a brave outlook when you have so much against you is admirable. They're the heroes.

# TWO KINDS OF PEOPLE IN THE WORLD

There are basically two kinds of people who directly affect your world: those who are helpful, and those who are in your way. There's the guy who sees you coming and holds the elevator doors open for you. Then, there's the guy who pretends not to see you and quickly pushes the CLOSE DOOR button to be on his way—leaving you behind.

Then there are the those who are a whole new level of in your way.

The vehicle coming at me had entered the parking lot through the exit driveway instead of the entrance driveway, completely blocking me from driving forward. Where are those tire-ripping spikes when you need them?

The female driver was youngish, sporting a red bandana headscarf, with one hand on the steering wheel while the other hand palmed her café-au-something-or-another beverage. Twitching back and forth was the head of a little mouse-faced dog that must have been sitting on her lap.

She ever so slightly angled her car away and motioned me to roll down my window. I obliged and awaited her apology for the faux pas. Instead, she commanded that I back up so she could get by. I responded by pointing out that she was in the wrong, had entered through the exit, and if she backed up about ten feet, we could both get out of this alive.

Bandana Head's eyes were devoid of acknowledgment. With a *blink, blink,* she palmed me with a talk-to-the-hand gesture and said, "I'm sensing some hostility here."

My frustration level went stratospheric. The temptation to let it pop was right there. Unwire the cork, and like a bottle of shaken champagne, unleash a firehose of expletives followed by a nuclear-grade-mushroom-cloud single-finger gesture of profanity. Bandana Head was like meat on a hook above the pack of hungry hounds, and I was the big dog. Yes, I wanted to let her have it. I wanted to reach through her mouth, rip out her spinal cord, and beat her with it.

I couldn't control or change the situation or escape the self-indulgent person in front of me, nor can I in any way ever, ever, ever control how people act. The one thing I did have control over was how I reacted. My reaction was 100 percent in my power.

I took a deep breath, backed up my car, and saved my sanity for the higher good.

**No one can make you feel inferior without your consent.**
—ELEANOR ROOSEVELT

There are rogue Bandana Heads who roam freely throughout our society inflicting judgment, turmoil, and criticism, and testing the

📌

Don't let negative people mess with your juju or penetrate your bubble. Reserve your mind for a higher level of thinking.

Before you argue with someone, ask yourself, are they open to a different perspective? If not, there's no point.

bounds of a person's compassionate limits. Engaging in or reacting to their annoying, poor, irritating behavior only brings you into the negativity tornado that is swirling around them. For the sake of your sanity, walk away. But if you're so compelled by their negative behavior to engage, choose your battles wisely.

Aristotle wrote, "Anyone can become angry—that is easy. But to become angry with the right person, to the right degree, at the right time, for the right purpose, and in the right way—that is* not easy."

## LONELINESS AND ISOLATION

The body sees loneliness and isolation as a mortal threat. "The mortality rate for air pollution is 5 percent. For loneliness, it's 25 percent." said John Cacioppo, director of the University of Chicago's Center for Cognitive and Social Neuroscience.[80]

Feeling loneliness is damaging to the body. Immune responses are suppressed, and inflammation becomes more prevalent, which fuels other diseases including cancers and Alzheimer's.

Steve Cole has studied biobehavioral science as professor at David Geffen School of Medicine at UCLA. In the early 2000s, a study revealed closeted gay men with HIV died much faster rate than gay men with HIV who were open about their sexuality.[81] The immune systems of the closeted gay men were poor in comparison to those of the men who were openly gay. If loneliness compromises the immune system of those closeted gay men to shorten their lives, then loneliness could turn any disease deadly.

Our culture is changing. We spend more time in isolated environments, on social media, binge-watching the thousands of readily available TV shows, and spending time on the computer rather than being with people. It's estimated over 20 percent of the population suffers the pain of loneliness. That number is expected to rise with the baby boomer population retiring. For boomers, their empty nests, their families dispersing to other cities, and the death of their friends and relatives only add more to their loneliness. Loneliness and its negative health consequences are on the way to a widespread cultural epidemic.

A broken heart is a broken heart. Lost love from marriages failing and from children, friends, and family moving away is painful, but its more than just the emotional pain. It turns out the brain registers loneliness with the same neural activity as physical pain. A broken heart is really painfully broken. We talk about rejection as hurting because it actually does hurt.

Social pain can be just as serious as physical pain. The cure is easy: turn off your cell phone and have a conversation. Stay connected. Being connected to others is important to our very survival.

Our psychological health is as important as our physical health. We spend billions of dollars on personal care items like deodorants, hair care products, dental floss, and arch support—but there's no aisle in the drugstore for mental health.

We fear failure, rejection, and loneliness. We ruminate over past mistakes and conflicts with others. We sometimes suffer psychological wounds that make us believe those around us care much less about us than they actually do. Sometimes we misinterpret someone not returning our call as a blatant rejection, while it may just be the person is dealing with issues of their own. Then we retreat for fear of further rejection.

Rejection or other emotional pain registers in the same place in the brain as physical pain. Because of this pain pathway, people who experience rejection are at greater risk of anger and aggression or dangerously lashing out, like a fired coworker "going postal" or bullied kids resorting to school shootings. Instead of anger, the best cure is to reach out to those who love us and who will comfort us.

We have such a need to belong to groups. Reaching out to those who care for us has been found to soothe the sting of rejection. Doing so is important as emotional pain has such a detrimental effect on our well-being.

A hug a day would be just what the doctor ordered—the healing power of a hug is real. Hugs help dissipate stress and negative emotions caused by interpersonal conflicts. Hugs calm your nervous system, lower your blood pressure and help relax your mood.

Good relationships, love, friendship, and connectedness keep us happier and healthier. No matter what we do, we need each other. People bring comfort, love, and someone to confide in. We have a sense of belonging. People help us achieve our goals and learn new skills. Stay connected—it's a lifesaver.

> *We're born alone, we live alone, we die alone. Only through our love and friendship can we create the illusion for the moment that we're not alone.*
> —ORSON WELLES

## ROSETO GROUP HUG—THE POWER OF THE CLAN

Around the middle of the twentieth century, and peaking in the mid-1960s, heart disease had become the most common cause of death. It's good to remember this was long before the FDA approved statins to help reduce the risk of heart disease. The first statin, lovastatin, wasn't approved until 1987, and widespread use didn't happen until the 1990s.

The dramatic increase in heart disease during the mid-twentieth century and into the 1960s was due to the increase in smoking and dietary changes that lead to increased serum cholesterol levels.[82] In contrast, at the beginning of the twentieth century, the most common cause of death was pneumonia and other infectious diseases. Heart disease was different; it was a disease caused by a lifestyle of smoking and poor diet.

The Roseto effect refers to a phenomenon that happened in Roseto, Pennsylvania, in the 1950s and '60s. The inhabitants of Roseto were not dying of any of the usual maladies plaguing society at that time—heart disease and diabetes—but instead were living well into old age. In particular, they had an extremely low incidence of heart disease, despite their voracious appetite for fat-heavy foods with sausages and meatballs fried in lard, wine, and unfiltered cigars and cigarettes. The men had hefty bodies, did backbreaking work in slate quarries that also added unsafe gases and dust to the air they inhaled. This Italian American town had the heart attack lifestyle that should have statistically put them higher than the national average, but instead was closer to nil.

Dr. Stewart Wolf, professor and medical director of the University of Oklahoma School of Medicine, had bought a farm in the Poconos region of Pennsylvania for a summer retreat. While he was having a few beers with the local doctor, the doctor mentioned that heart disease seemed far less common in Roseto, even compared to the neighboring town of Bangor where mostly non-Italians lived. This ignited intrigue in Wolf and led him to investigate the phenomenon. Why was Roseto, populated by Italian-Americans, different from neighboring towns?

Over four years, the adults of Roseto were thoroughly examined and interviewed, and their diets were scrutinized. Comparisons were made with two nearby towns, and in 1966 Wolf and his colleague, sociologist John G. Bruhn, co-authored their findings in the *Journal of the American Medical Association*. Baffling as it was, the data only ruled out genetic or any other sources for the dilemma.

Wolf then looked beyond the data to the community and discovered two clues: there was no crime, and public assistance was zero. Wolf started looking closer at the family structure and found there to typically be three generations under one roof and the elderly were revered in the community. People stopped and said hello as they traveled down the street. There were community rituals, social clubs, and church festivals, and the ideal of village life was pervasive. Wolf took notice.

Wolf's conclusion was the answers didn't lie in the research or statistics, but in the spirit and connectedness. The community support, that sense of belonging, love, unfailing joyous attitude, and family life ruled the community and were the key in Roseto inhabitants living long lives.

#### *People are nourished by other people.*
−DR. STEWART WOLF, AMERICAN PHYSICIAN AND RESEARCHER

Roseto did not happen by chance, but by their roots.

At the beginning of the twentieth century, 85 percent of Italian immigrants came from the southern region of Calabria in Italy. In 1860, Giuseppe Garibaldi forced out the Bourbons invaders from the country for good and united poorer southern Italy with the more prosperous north. The problem was northern Italy did nothing for their southern peasants. Instead they imposed heavy taxes on them.

Most southern peasants could barely survive, especially when the government taxed everything. If the government knew you had a cow, mule or garden, then you would be taxed accordingly. Families started hiding their livestock and gardens. Everyone in authority became the enemy, and family became the one thing that could be trusted. No one could be trusted outside the family or close friends, and families were forced into privacy. Immigrants brought the idea of trusting only those within the family with them to the United States.

Most of the original settlers of Roseto, Pennsylvania came from Roseto, Valfortore in the province of Foggia, and undoubtedly faced the same pressures of their fellow southern Italians. Starting in the 1880s, the first small group sailed to America and eventually found work in the slate mines of Pennsylvania. Word went back, and over the next decade or so, the small Italian village of Roseto, Valfortore was abandoned. In 1894, twelve hundred immigrants came to an area outside of Bangor, Pennsylvania to start their new life in a new town they called Roseto.

When they came to the United States, they brought their *paesani* culture with them. This unbreakable bond of trust, family, and friends prevailed.

Settling in Pennsylvania had its problems, and the early immigrants of Roseto were shunned by those who dominated the area, the English and Welsh. The Rosetans turned inward again, to their community and culture.

In *The Power of Clan*, Wolf and Bruhn observe:

"What has been learned seems to confirm an old but often forgotten conviction that mutual respect and cooperation contribute to the health and welfare of a community and its inhabitants, and that self-indulgence and lack of concern for others exert opposite influences."

"We looked at the social structures of healthy communities," Wolf concluded, "and found that they are characterized by stability and pre-dictability. In those communities, each person has a clearly defined role in the social scheme.[83]

Wolf explained that an isolated individual might be overwhelmed by the problems of everyday life. Such a person internalizes that feeling as stress which, in turn, can adversely affect everything from blood pressure to kidney function. That's less likely an outcome when a person is surrounded by caring friends, neighbors, and relatives. The sense of being supported reduces stress, and the burdens of diseases.

> *When you come from a big family, you see that,*
> *growing up, you're learning how to share. Your sisters*
> *have got your back; "You're not alone in this—we all*
> *support you!" Your family provides that, it gives you*
> *a sense of safety, and it's a very grounding feeling.*
> —GISELE BUNDCHEN, SUPERMODEL

## BESTIES ARE THE BEST

Best friends have your back, and make you a better person. They're a form of soulmate and someone to share everything with. They're your rock. And vice-versa.

In July 1848, in Seneca Falls, New York, the first Women's Rights Con-vention was held to discuss the condition of rights of women. At that time, most women had no right to own property. They were banned from attending almost all colleges. If divorced, were not entitled custody of their children. And did not have control of their own bodies to choose not to have more children. They could not keep the wages they earned—that money belonged to their husbands—or serve on a jury. They certainly had no right to vote to change any of these egregious laws.

Women were deemed to be the chattel of their husbands in all manners, including sexually, and were obliged to obey laws they had taken no part in creating. If by a miracle there was a divorce, women were entitled to no more than the clothing on their backs and absolutely no rights to their own children.

It was Elizabeth Cady Stanton who addressed the crowd at the first Women's Rights Convention, but she was soon joined by Susan B. Anthony. The two spent the rest of their lives together as allies and adversaries, forging history and friendship.

"I forge the thunderbolts, and she fired them," said Elizabeth Cady Stanton of Susan B. Anthony. "Best friends should be more like a thorn in your side than an echo of your own thoughts," said Anthony of her friend Stanton.

*God grant me the serenity to accept the things*
*I cannot change, courage to change the things*
*I can, and wisdom to know the difference.*
—REINHOLD NIEBUHR, THEOLOGIAN, THE SERENITY PRAYER

Being married and a mother to seven children, Elizabeth Cady Stanton was an unlikely crusader. Elizabeth was homebound, raising her children, and had little time to change the world. It was her life-long friendship and support of her dear friend, Susan B. Anthony, that put the legs to her ideas in the world. Although she had suitors, Susan B. Anthony never married. Marriage may have compromised her independence and her work to change women's rights. Nothing could stand in her way to attain the same freedoms and empowerments known only to men at that time.

In a time when women did not travel alone—that would have been scandalous—Susan knew the train schedules by heart. She traveled throughout the United States and Europe, giving approximately one hundred speeches a year. She continued to do so for almost fifty years, spreading the notion that women need to stand on their own as equals in this world, and have their own self-worth.

In 1906, at the age of eighty-six, Susan B. Anthony died. Since the first Women's Rights Convention in Seneca Falls, she had spent fifty-eight years fighting for a woman's right to vote. On November 2, 1920, eight million women stepped forward and cast their votes in a presidential election for the first time. Finally, women could put a portion of their own destiny in their own hands—thanks in large part to the friendship of these two incredible women.[84]

You don't need a certain number of friends, just a number of friends you can be certain of.

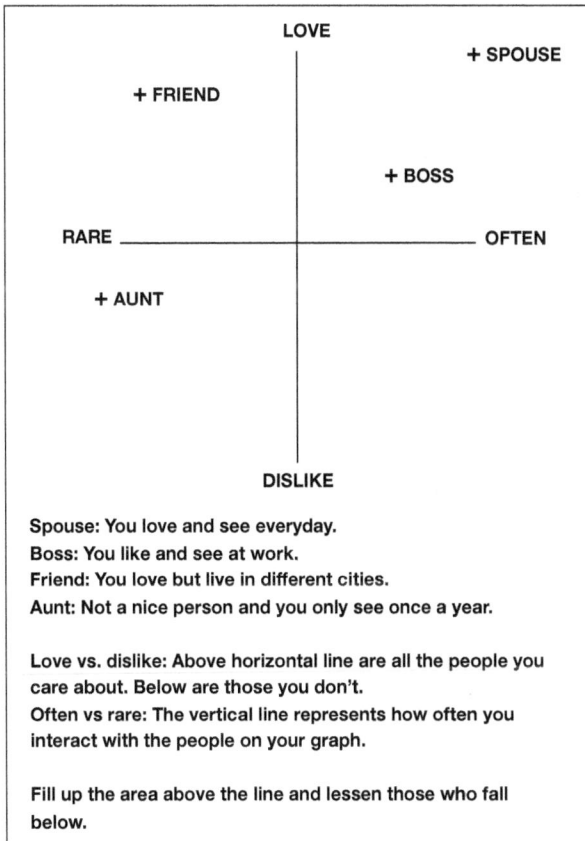

```
                        LOVE
                               + SPOUSE
              + FRIEND

                               + BOSS

      RARE _____|_____ OFTEN

          + AUNT




                        DISLIKE
```

Spouse: You love and see everyday.
Boss: You like and see at work.
Friend: You love but live in different cities.
Aunt: Not a nice person and you only see once a year.

Love vs. dislike: Above horizontal line are all the people you care about. Below are those you don't.
Often vs rare: The vertical line represents how often you interact with the people on your graph.

Fill up the area above the line and lessen those who fall below.

# GRAY AREA—LOVE VS. HATE

Spending time on the beautiful Indonesian island of Bali, you'll soon notice that black-and-white checkered cloth is draped everywhere. You see it wrapped around guardian statues in front of puras or temples, worn by dancers in ceremonies, or hung around the gates of shrines, even around trees. The black and white cloth, known as a saput poleng, is used in the Hindu religion and culturally in Bali to represent the extreme contradictions found in all aspects of life.

Life is full of opposition such as happiness and sadness, and then there's the entire spectrum between these two opposites. This concept of duality doesn't stop with just emotions. It goes for everything. If there's night, then there's day, yin and yang, rich and poor, high and low, good and evil, right and wrong, and so on.

The Balinese culture recognizes that life is very complicated and full of polar opposites or contradictions. Sorrow is part of happiness. Enlightenment may come through an inner reflection of past mistakes. All polar opposites are equally embraced as the truths the Balinese find in life. We only know what's right when we see what's wrong. The most profound truth is that between the black and white of everything lies the gray area.

The Balinese saput poleng is a traditional pattern with one strip of black threads, then one strip of an equal number of white threads, both vertically and horizontally. It produces four checked segments, one square of pure black and one of pure white and two squares of gray, the mix of the black and white threads. This may be a simplified interpretation of humanity as a whole, translating the thread patterns into human nature as 25 percent white, or good; 25 percent black, or evil; and the remaining 50 percent is the gray area.

We're taught to believe that when it comes to good and evil, evil will be defeated and good will prevail. But as the Balinese point out in the equal parts of both black and white areas in the cloth, we as humans are thoroughly and equally capable of following both directions. Good doesn't always and will not always prevail. Humans are equally capable of both great acts of kindness as well as despicable acts.

There are people who are brutes and people who are good Samaritans. There are both Mother Teresa and Jeffery Dahmer. How do two such polar opposite qualities exist in our humanity? The dichotomy of good and evil seems like it would be easy to pinpoint as they are complete opposites.

For example, evil would be killing someone. But killing someone for God or your country swings the pendulum from evil to good. The ironic problem is there are many different gods and many different countries. Who's right? Who's wrong? In life, it's the gray area that wins out more than black and white.

In the movie *American Sniper*, Bradley Cooper portrays US Navy Seal sharpshooter Chris Kyle, the most lethal sniper in American history. He served four tours of duty in Iraq with 160 confirmed kills, although the number of kills is not officially declared by the US military. He received two Silver Star Medals, five Bronze Star Medals, one Navy and Marine Corps Commendation Medal, two Navy and Marine Corps Achievement Medals and numerous other unit and personal awards. Whether the script is reality or not, in the movie, Kyle felt he was good with his God and country for his actions.[85]

The Iraqi insurgents nicknamed Chris Kyle the Devil of Ramadi, but the Iraqis had their own devil shooting right back at the US troops. Juba was a sniper with a Sunni insurgent group in the Islamic Army of Iraq. Around 2006, Juba claimed to have killed more than 143 US service-members. War is a conflict to the death, and whether you're right or wrong depends on which side you fight.[86]

The polar opposite would be peace, a state of affairs the world has rarely seen on a consistent basis. The deadliest war in history for cumulative number of deaths is the Second World War, with sixty to eighty-five million fatalities, followed by the Mongol conquests, between 1206 and 1337, with a death toll of more than forty-one million over a hundred-plus-year period.

The duality exists between love and hate. Knowing this will helps us understand that in humanity, there's always a choice as to which direction you want to go. We often easily choose love, but in those times when you feel the hate rising, you must remember it's your choice as to how you want to proceed.

> *Find joy in everything you choose to do.*
> *Every job, relationship, home ... It's your*
> *responsibility to love it, or change it.*
> —CHUCK PALAHNIUK, AMERICAN NOVELIST

## TURNING CONFLICT TO PEACE

Conflict is created when there are two opposing sides of thought. Two people or two groups of people are at opposition, and both sides are trying to move the other to their way of thinking. The conflict is we want the opposition to see we're right, they're wrong, jump on our bandwagon, and think the way we think. The problem with I'm right, you're wrong, is it sets up each side to only be after a win. There's no room for compromise or negotiation.

Instead, what if we didn't focus so hard on proving the other side wrong or only going for an all-out win? How about having the courage and humility to learn why the opposition has their view? Your brain learns only when it's open and moves to understanding rather than chastising. With the curiosity to learn from each other, to seek understanding instead of chastising, and with a sense of compassion, we can open up the situation for discussion and compromise.

Everyone comes to the table with a different viewpoint. Give each other the kindness to hear what that viewpoint is and to understand.

## ACTS OF KINDNESS

In the presence of something good, the brain releases four main feel-good chemicals. As we've touched on already, dopamine, serotonin, oxytocin and endorphins are associated with feelings of happiness, euphoria, and bliss, as well as with motivation and concentration. Acts of kindness can release hormones that elevate your mood and overall well-being. That warm and fuzzy feeling is your brain chemistry at work.

The release of dopamine is linked with random acts of kindness. Oxytocin plays a role in forming trust in people and social bonds. For our species to survive we had to work together and form communities and bonds. Our ancestral brain is hardwired to be altruistic and help one another. When we see someone in distress or a child in trouble, our instinct is to help before we can even think about it. Even if we put our own life in peril, our instinct overrides our reason, and we spring into action.

When acts of kindness and feelings of gratitude literally flood our brains with dopamine, serotonin and oxytocin, it creates a natural happiness high. Giving and kindness are a powerful pathway for creating joy in ourselves, elevating our mood, and improving our overall health.

It's the little things that really add up. No matter how big or how small, each act of kindness has an impact on those we helped and on ourselves. It's a gift that boomerangs back to you.

*Too often we underestimate the power of a touch, a smile, a kind word, a listening ear, an honest compliment, or the smallest act of caring, all of which have the potential to turn a life around.*

—LEO BUSCAGLIA, AUTHOR KNOWN AS "DR. LOVE"

## GRATITUDE

Keith Richards, cofounder of the Rolling Stones, has had a very long career at the top of rock stardom. The band was formed in 1962, and Richards is the lead guitarist as well as contributing vocalist and songwriter. *Rolling Stone* magazine called Richards the creator of "rock's greatest single body of riffs" on the guitar."[87]

During the 1960s and 1970s, Richards was busted for drugs five times and openly admitted to using heroin and other substances. Throughout the years, he's experienced drug troubles, arrests, jail time—the list goes on—then miraculously went back to being a rock god performing on stage and touring the world.

Born in 1943, and still performing today, Richards may not be riding the drug-crazy days anymore. He's certainly raised enough hell for several lifetimes. With over fifty years in the limelight, he has mellowed and as he looks back on his career and life, he sums it up with, "It's great to be here, it's great to be anywhere."

Maybe you didn't test life like Keith Richards, but you're still here. Being grateful. Waking up every day and giving thanks you're even here. It's a great way to start the day, to say yourself, I'm glad to be here.

Gratitude is a warm feeling created from thankfulness. Scientific evidence shows that expressing genuine gratitude on a daily basis can improve your overall health and your physiological functions. Gratitude is associated with better sleep, improved digestion, reduced aches and pains, and reduced stress, and grateful people generally take better care of themselves. Being contented, thankful or pleased are all within your own power. It's a practice. Something to incorporate into your daily routine.

**Gratitude is the solution to anger and fear.**
—TONY ROBBINS, MOTIVATIONAL SPEAKER

## CHAPTER SUMMARY

☑ Stay connected to people, not things.

☑ Be involved with your community, your church, or an organization.

☑ Send love into the world and be open to receiving it.

☑ Begin the day by expressing gratitude.

☑ Do a small random act of kindness every day.

☑ Listen to any song by the Rolling Stones.

## CHAPTER TWELVE

# Intelligence

*There are three kinds of men. The one that learns by reading. The few who learn by observation. The rest of them have to pee on the electric fence for themselves.*

—WILL ROGERS

This quote, often attributed to Will Rogers, is one of my favorites. It brings back memories of my youth. If you're not sure what this quote means, read on.

Will Rogers was born in 1879—he thought so, anyway. They didn't always keep accurate birth records back then. Born on a ranch in the Indian Territory of Oklahoma, he was part Cherokee. He quipped that his ancestors didn't come over on the *Mayflower*, but being from American Indian descendants, they "met the boat."

He turned his cowboy abilities and humor into a vaudeville cowboy rope act that led him to the *Ziegfeld Follies* Broadway production. Then he went on to become one of the most popular, highest-paid film stars of the 1920s and 1930s. He wrote more than four thousand nationally syndicated newspaper columns, making him, his humor, and his philosophies popular with Americans of all walks of life. He downplayed academia, noting, "Everybody is ignorant, only on different subjects."[88]

We're all ignorant about something.

Will Roger's quote about electric fences brings back memories as a young girl visiting my uncle's farm in Topeka, Kansas. For those of you who haven't been on a farm or herded cattle, electric fences are used to keep the cows from wandering into another pasture. If touched, it gives a stunning shock. Back then, I remember my older brother convincing my younger brother to pee on the electric fence. If the shock of the electric fence needed to be strong enough to move a cow, you can imagine what it might have done to my little brother's wiener!

My older brother was adamant, yelling, "Don't be a baby! It doesn't hurt!" He was taunting my little brother to do it. Initially, it didn't sound like a good idea to me but my older brother was so insistent and convincing. Convincing to the point that I wondered, If I could have shot pee in a specific direction, would I have succumbed to by my older brother's enthusiasm and peed on the fence too?

This is when adult supervision would have been a good idea. But my little brother zipped down his pants, pointed, peed, and suffered the consequences of a shocking experience.

It made no sense to pee on an electric fence, but my little brother did it anyway. Why?

## SWAYING REALITY

*Brainshift* is a phenomenon where our subconscious shifts our perception and contradicts objective reality, distorting what we see, hear, and know. It's not related to our intelligence, morals or past experiences. We don't know it's even happening. At the moment, we do things that seem okay, but that most likely appear foolish to others. It happens under sets of conditions that cause us to do regrettable things contrary to our rational beliefs.

It occurs in two distinct situations: those involving high anxiety, and those associated with major reward.[89]

My little brother was in a high-anxiety situation. He was being taunted by my older brother not to be a sissy and do it. For a little kid, this is probably one of the most stressful situations. Live up to your older brother's challenge or be labeled a wussy. Deeply he probably knew nothing good could come from peeing on an electric fence, but his logical thinking left, and the high anxiety of the situation made him do it. No matter the consequences—an electric shock to his wiener—the taunting and stress would be over.

In the next two sections—peer pressure and the temptation of an overwhelming advantage—I discuss the two situations in more details. Whether it is a high-anxiety situation or one associated with major rewards, the phenomenon of Brainshift can lead us astray.

## PEER PRESSURE

What other people say has an impact on how we proceed, what we see, how we decide, and how we might answer a question. It's the need for social conformity. We usually cave under group pressure, especially when the group is adamant and overwhelming.

An interesting study on peer pressure was done in the 1950s by Dr. Solomon Asch. The subjects were shown cards that had lines drawn on them. The test participants were to choose lines with matching lengths. Pretty straightforward, something a five-year-old could do in a heartbeat.

The twist was seven of the eight test participants were in cahoots with Dr. Asch, stooges set up to fool the one real participant. The stooges were directed to choose an incorrect answer. Each person had to state aloud their answers, so when it got to the lone real participant, he had a choice to make. Go with what his eyes were telling him and choose the right answer, or conform with the group and choose incorrectly.

On average, 32 percent, approximately a third of the real participants, choose wrongly on the first go-around. The experiment was repeated many times with the same real participants, and over 75 percent eventually caved and conformed with the group. Only 25 percent never conformed.[90]

You're probably thinking, I would never do that! I would never conform.

Really?

Dr. Asch wondered about his findings. Did social pressure change their perception? Was it all just about fitting in?

The conclusion was twofold. First, we cave. Yes, we want to fit in—the social pressure can be enormous. Second, we sometimes feel the wisdom of the crowd is better, that a majority represents a better collective or wiser choice.[91]

There's truth in the crowd being wiser. Research has shown the group's opinion is often more accurate than the opinion of a single individual of the group. *The Wisdom of Crowds* author James Surowiecki highlights numerous case studies where the crowd's opinion was better and more accurate than any single opinion.

For example, at a county fair people were asked to guess the weight of an ox. No single guess was as accurate as the average of all the guesses. The aggregation of the crowd's opinion played an important role in accuracy. The aggregation of the crowd's opinion played an important role in accuracy, both in this specific circumstance and in general. For this reason, we sometimes go along with the opinion of the crowd as being more accurate than our own.

In Dr. Asch's study, choosing matching lines had no significant conse-
quence for the future of the participants' lives. Nothing substantial was
at risk. Nothing was lost or gained. What difference did it make? Even
so, it's good to understand that the crowd's momentum can and does
affect our behavior.

The influence of the crowd can easily alter our point of view. We adopt
behaviors, buy merchandise, and follow trends based on the cues set
by the crowd.

Ever go to a Major League Baseball game? The crowd is pumped for
their home team. People are buying hats, keychains and jerseys with
the names of their favorite players, and the next thing you know—you're
wearing a giant foam hand gesturing number one. You had no plans
to buy a foam glove that would fit a giant. It has no useful purpose
when you get home—but at the time, the energy of the crowd has you
buying giant foam hands, eating nachos out of a plastic baseball cap,
and drinking beer from a tube going to the beer bong hat on your head.

The crowd mentality at a baseball game can be fun. Being part of the
excitement is rewarding, but a crowd can turn ugly and have a darker
side. Under the right circumstances, the crowd can become a mob.

When the wisdom of the crowd turns ugly, it becomes a mob mentality.
Our identity disappears simply by being part of the mob, and we lose our
sense of responsibility. Mob-mentality behavior is mostly influenced by
anonymity—you become one among the many. When the mob mentality
carries us along, we get caught up in doing things contrary to our natures
or beliefs, things that are usually detrimental to ourselves or others.

Choosing matching lines has insignificant outcomes. But when the
stakes are higher, would we still cave? When the wisdom of the crowd
turns dark to a mob mentality, truth itself is in serious jeopardy. It's why
we have jury trials—to find the truth.

The accuracy of the wisdom of the crowd can be useful when formulating public policy, identifying social norms, or guessing the weight of an ox. The crowd can also be fun, like at baseball games, but it can also turn ugly. When it's bad, the crowd becomes a mindless mob that has gone from innocent participant to people pushing a more sinister outcome.

## THE TEMPTATION OF AN OVERWHELMING ADVANTAGE

There's another type of situation that can have us doing things we know are wrong. When a situation involves high rewards, the temptation to get those rewards can cause us to make bad, selfish decisions. We're vulnerable to get-rich-quick schemes. Our desires for money, cutting corners to get what we want, buying our way in, sex, fame, and recognition are intoxicating and sometimes irresistible.

Sometimes, we try to justify self-indulgent, bad behavior. Ignoring certain facts and instead only presenting only the information that supports and defends our actions in an attempt to somehow prove we're right. This is called *anchoring*.

For example, when the consequences are high, like jail time or losing an expensive court case, we don't want to admit we're wrong. We then build our story, finding data to defend our actions and fit the decisions we've already made. After all, the court system gives us the baseline of being presumed innocent until proven guilty.

Lori Laughlin, famed actress for her TV role on *Full House*, and her husband, Mossimo Giannulli, stand accused of paying five hundred thousand dollars in bribes to get their two daughters into the University of Southern California, one of California's most prestigious universities. The two daughters were admitted as athletic recruits to the USC rowing team. The fact that neither one has ever rowed on a crew boat may have been a key factor in the prosecution forming the allegation of bribery.

Laughlin and Giannulli's defense? The money was a donation to the university, not a bribe.

What were they thinking?

Maybe they weren't thinking or asking themselves, What's wrong with this picture? How can our two daughters, who have no rowing experience, be recruits for the USC rowing team? Now that they've been charged with a crime, they are sticking to their story that it was only a donation.

Maybe the enticement of a high reward, getting their daughters into a prestigious university, outweighed their ability to make a rational, unbiased, ethical decision. The high reward changed their perception of reality. And now, they're *anchored* in their belief they did nothing wrong and have built a defense to support their claim that it was a donation, not a bribe. Maybe their hot-shot defense team will be able to prove the donation technically was not related to their daughters being crew recruits and be exonerated from all charges. The case is yet to be determined.

According to the US legal principle of presumption of innocence, the prosecution must present compelling evidence—the legal burden of proof—that proves the accused is guilty. The same is true for this case that is still pending at the time of writing this book.

Like a moth to the flame—fame, fortune, or some other high reward—we get mesmerized into doing things we normally would think are wrong. Our normal behaviors or belief are overridden with by temptation causing us to do things inconsistent with our fundamental ways. Then through self-justification, we can go so far as to deny any negative feedback associated with those thoughts or actions.

It's important to admit our mistakes—it's a vital tool for learning and personal development. It's painful, sometimes too painful, which is why we'll go to great lengths to revise, negotiate, and convince ourselves and others that we're right. The mirror held up to look at our mistakes is sometimes just too much to look at.

We are possibly hardwired to lie to ourselves. On an honesty scale of 1 to 10, most of us probably think we're a 7 or above. We give ourselves top marks for positive traits. We overestimate everything from our looks to our IQ. This phenomenon is known as *illusory superiority*, and it's so prevalent that we can honestly say we're all guilty.

A study revealed 94 percent of the professors at a university rated themselves above average relative to their peers. In another study, 32 percent of the employees of a software company said they performed better than nineteen out of twenty of their colleagues. Overestimating our abilities may help support our mental health and build our self-confidence. The illusion of overvaluing our skills may be a protective measure to shield our self-esteem, and that's good for a positive mental outlook.[92]

However, in the case of those trying to scam the system, leapfrog ahead, or give themselves an overwhelming advantage, their overconfidence may lead them to believe they deserve to be treated better because they think they are better. One way to curb the self-indulgence is to focus on self-improvement. Don't believe you are better than everyone else, but focus on becoming the best version of you.

## PROCRASTINATION: PRESENT SELF VS. FUTURE SELF

We tend to value immediate rewards more than future rewards. When you think of your future goals, you're making plans for your Future Self. Meanwhile, it's your Present Self who has to do all the hard work to attain those goals. Your Present Self has to set out guidelines and make progress for your Future Self to achieve your desires.

The big hiccup is we live in the present with the Present Self, and the Present Self may want to do a hundred other things instead of the work to make the Future Self happy. Present Self wants to go to the friend's party tonight, but Future Self wants Present Self to finish the tax return by tomorrow morning. The Future Self can be a killjoy for the Present Self's fun.[93]

Procrastination has levels. Putting off doing the laundry means you won't have a clean shirt tomorrow. That's not a biggie. Putting off finishing your degree to get the promised promotion and more money is a biggie. I have one philosophy against procrastination. How long can you afford to put off the person you want to be? Hold yourself accountable by regularly asking yourself, What do I genuinely, sincerely aspire to have, do, and become? Do I have a solid goal? What am I doing today to accomplish that goal? Awareness will keep you on track.

I was able to finish this book by holding myself accountable. I logged my progress by how many words I'd written towards my goal of completion.

Then I enlisted my trainer. We had training sessions twice a week and between squats I would report how many words I had written for the week. It became a regular topic through our sessions. We talked about number of pages, content, and what was happening next. He was my captive audience holding me accountable for fitness and for completing the book, a double whammy. Many studies show the huge benefits of an accountability buddy and letting others know your goals. When I got up to about 20,000 words, I started blabbing to my close friends that I was writing a book. By doing this, it made me commit even more—no matter what, I had to finish now. My pride was at stake. Enlisting the encouragement of my circle of friends, the people I saw on a regular basis, held me even more accountable. By announcing my goals to the world, my goal was no longer lounging on the Someday Isle. It was now. Completing the book was made doable through accountability.

Commitment and accomplishing daily tasks will lead to achieving life goals.

I have a funny analogy about accomplishing tasks: Picture a task as a toothache. Your tooth hurts. It's very sensitive, and you figure you probably need a root canal for the pain to go completely away. When do you want your root canal? As soon as possible, or way in the future? When do you want the pain to be over? Difficult tasks are like toothaches: it's better to get them over sooner rather than later.

In the meantime, we worry over future deadlines we know we need to meet. You can take the worry, frustration, and pain out of it by creating a plan to get the work done. As they say, failing to plan is planning to fail. Doing the work is not the problem—it's usually starting it. So stop procrastinating by starting the work or scheduling it to be completed before it becomes a problem. Set a goal of fifteen-minutes increments. At the end of fifteen minutes, see how much you've done. Chances are you've built the momentum you need to continue. Breaking it down is key, or as the saying goes, "It's harder by the yard, but a cinch by the inch."

One of the reasons we procrastinate is we're afraid of failing at the task. Failure hurts, and the best way to avoid the pain of failure is to procrastinate. Our deep-seated logic makes us disinclined to take on the project or finish it. Procrastination then becomes comforting as an alternative to failure.

Understand mistakes happen, and most are not all that bad. Generally, failure can be a stepping-stone to greatness. When it came to inventing the light bulb, Thomas Edison famously said, "I have not failed, I've just found ten thousand ways that it won't work."

## CONSEQUENCES OF BAD HABITS

Making a mistake is one thing—as we've already said, humans are subject to error. We're not perfect.

Aside from the results of our mistakes, negative consequences can also be the result of having bad habits or behaviors, but there are degrees to consider as to how bad is bad.

Bad habits come in sizes—from small ones we can live with to larger-than-life ones that can cause physical and emotional damage. A not-so-bad habit is a behavior that, with a little effort, we could change or stop altogether. Behaviors that interfere with the quality of our lives are problematic obstacles to our Future Self and success.

Ask yourself: Is my behavior of [name behavior here] an obstacle to my future success and well-being?

> **Good or bad, habits always deliver results.**
> —JACK CANFIELD, AUTHOR

Biting your nails is a small, relatively innocuous bad habit. It won't kill you, but it's considered unhealthy, as hands pick up germs from the things we touch. Also, it's not as attractive as having well-kept, manicured nails. Still it's not a severe detriment to your future success or overall health, and well-being.

Nail-biting is a small level of addiction because you're doing it repeatedly, maybe even mindlessly, or as a nervous tic. With a little effort, it's something within your control to address and stop. It's not activated by or dependent on the presence of an outside influence or substance. You don't have to dip your fingers in chocolate to get you to chew at your nails.

Small bad habits, like biting your nails, picking at your hair, staying up too late, eating donuts for breakfast, or watching too much television are habits that can be altered by changing your behaviors. It may be uncomfortable at first, but with some effort, it's doable. It's up to you and what you'll do about them, though.

That's the issue with small bad habits. They still take an effort to change. You can't blame them on anyone or anything but yourself. Letting small bad habits go on takes no energy, and that's where we get stuck. Making the effort takes effort.

When Admiral William H. McRaven said, "If you want to change the world, start off by making your bed," he was talking about building increments of pride in the choices you make every day, all day long until they become embedded, mindless positive habits.

The immediate reward of making your bed is a small sense of pride that'll give you the boost you need to move onto the next task, and then the next. It's the little things in life that matter.

> **If you can't do the little things right,**
> **you'll never be able to do the big things right.**
> —ADMIRAL WILLIAM H. MCRAVEN

For every action, there's an outcome or immediate reward. But repeated daily, these actions become habits, and habits become your life, with long-term negative or positive consequences.

Eating donuts for breakfast gives the immediate pleasure that sugary foods offer, but eating them every day could lead to weight gain and long-term, harmful health consequences such as insulin resistance or diabetes.

As I said, biting your nails could just be an occasional nervous tic or it could be worse. Nail-biting has been associated with a way to release

📌

You can't escape the consequences of your daily decisions. Making small, positive, healthy choices will serve you well long-term. It's more doable and easier than you think. It doesn't matter how slow you move as long as you move toward the positive.

anxiety. On a long-term basis this habit exposes you to more bacteria, possibly leading to infection around the nails, and over time, could be a contributing factor to a larger impulse disorder.

The disconnect between the short-term and long-term consequences of our actions is the hiccup. We're not thinking ahead, or we don't want to think ahead as the immediate short-term effect is comforting and is all we're looking for or feel we can handle at that time.

A hit of cocaine has an immediate effect of elation and euphoria, but long-term use could very well be a cocaine addiction. One mistaken night of cocaine use is a few days of regret; cocaine addiction is a big, deep hole that you have to dig your way out of.

## THE STUPID SHIT WE DO

There are a few situations that are usually the cause for our development of harmful or bad habits. It can be a way we deal with stress or anxiety, like biting your nails or on occasion drinking too much alcohol. It can be a way of relieving boredom, like watching too much television or checking social media every five minutes.

Stress, boredom, and anxiety are not avoidable. The challenge is to handle these unpleasant emotions in a healthy, productive manners. If you're stressed or want to relieve anxiety, do something positive for the body.

Meditate, breathe, stretch, exercise, take a walk, or do whatever else you can think of that is a positive behavior. Boredom may be alleviated by sparking your curiosity in learning a new skill. Walk around a bookstore or library to get ideas for ways to occupy your time or discover a new hobby.

These same emotions—stress, anxiety, and boredom—can lead us to alleviate them in ways that are detrimental to our future selves, such as by using drugs or alcohol. When it comes to bad decisions and altered states of minds, here's the truth—given the right amounts of drugs and or alcohol, you're bound to do almost anything. That includes stupid shit. Sometimes really stupid life-damaging shit.

AWOL is a military term that means "absent without leave," or more fully, absent from one's post without the intent to desert or permission to leave. With drugs and alcohol, your brain goes AWOL. Your rational thinking has left your brain without your explicit consent.

Drugs and alcohol can mess you up and will derail your momentum in life like nothing else. Most people try drugs because they're bored, curious, stressed and anxious, or just wanting to feel good. As we've mentioned, drugs cause the brain to fire up those feel-good chemicals. The problem is the feel-good part of your brain gets used to them and needs more and more to attain a similar high. It's the same with alcohol. Then the aftermath of withdrawal can leave you miserable. Anyone who has had a severe hangover knows this is true.

Drug use may have started as a way to temporarily escape the boredom and stress of life, but if continued, it can quickly make your life much worse than imaginable. Nancy Reagan may have taken a simplistic approach in her "Just Say No" drug-free campaign, but if you had just said no in the beginning—day one, it would have made an enormous difference. A few days of regret for a drunken weekend versus a lifetime battle of fighting an addiction. What if you never took the chance?

## WELCOME TO THE STUPID ZONE

The Stupid zone is about bad behaviors. It has nothing to do with the intelligence you were born with or the lack of it. We are all have different talents or lack of them. That's not your fault or what this section is about.

Stupidity: behavior that shows a lack of good sense or judgement.

The stupid zone is different. We're all guilty of occasionally doing stupid things—or behavior. Calling someone stupid is harsh and insulting, and not what this section is about. Please remember that and take the following to only be about our behaviors.

In this section, we'll discover Carlo M Cipollo's hypothesis on stupidity, but please put your political correctness on hold and go with the concept that stupid people are people who do stupid things.

### *Stupid is as stupid does.*
−FORREST GUMP

In the movie, *Forrest Gump*, several times the main character is asked if he is stupid. Forrest's reply, "Stupid is as stupid does," means people should not be judged by their appearances but by their actions. Stupidity is based on deeds, that one's actions indicate one's level of stupidity or intelligence. Basically, you are what you do—it's about your behavior, your actions.

Carlo M. Cipolla was an Italian economic historian who theorized about a controversial subject: stupidity. In an essay, *The Basic Laws of Human Stupidity*, Mr. Cipolla posited that stupid people share certain traits, and there are more stupid people than we think. They're irrational. They cause problems. They lower society's well-being. Most importantly, there's no defense against the havoc they wreak, and the rest of us are left cleaning up their mess. Cipolla came up with five basic laws of human stupidity:[94]

**Law 1: "Always and inevitably, everyone underestimates the number of stupid individuals in circulation."**
Everyone underestimates the quantity of stupid people roaming around in society. We have a biased assumption that people who are well-educated, have impressive jobs or enjoy a certain status are also smart, but that is a presumption that Cipolla says is surprisingly false.

**Law 2: "The probability that a certain person will be stupid is independent of any other characteristic of that person."**
Every imaginable category of society has its fair share of stupid people. Gender, race, nationality, education, income or whether you work on Wall Street or main street makes no difference. Stupid people are a fixed constant across all populations, nations and areas of work. Cipolla didn't give an exact percentage for any categories, claiming any guess would violate his first law.

**Law 3: "A stupid person is a person who causes losses to another person or to a group of persons while himself deriving no gain and even possibly incurring losses."**
Here's is where Cipolla's laws strikes a nerve. A stupid person is one who causes problems for others without any clear benefit to himself and often to his own detriment.

Think of the classic story of the politician who spent campaign finances on his mistress. It makes no sense that the politician, who presumably has worked hard to get to where he is, would jeopardize his future. But this story and stories like it are all too familiar. Welcome to the Stupid Zone.

I have another great example, recently on the news a man stole a fire department ambulance from the scene of an accident. The area was surrounded by police and firemen working on the car crash and the victims involved. Yet Mr. Stupid must have thought this an ideal situation to steal the ambulance. Needless to say, a car chase ensued with dozens of police units. Mr. Stupid rammed cars along the street, plowed through a police car blockade, drove through fenced areas and wreaked havoc before he was cornered by more police cars and finally gave up.

What was Mr. Stupid thinking? Not only did he do great harm to others, he did great harm to himself. This is a perfect example of a person deep in the stupid zone. He put others in great peril and destroyed thousands of dollars in property, and his actions were detrimental to himself and most assuredly will result in jail time.

His actions were detrimental to society and the rest of us are left with cleaning up the mess.

**Law 4: "Non-stupid people always underestimate the damaging power of stupid individuals."**
Non-stupid people sometimes forget that stupid people are stupid. Non-stupid people forget that in any circumstance, dealing with a stupid person will usually turn out to be a mistake and often a costly mistake. Non-stupid people are going about their lives, thinking everyone is working like they are and doing their best—but that's where non-stupid people make the mistake. Stupid people usually are not focused on doing their best.

**Law 5: "A stupid person is the most dangerous type of person."**
Stupid people consistently make stupid choices that wreak havoc on society. Societies have to progress in spite of the this.

To illustrate stupidity better, Cipolla devised a graph with four sections divided by two axes. One axis is based on whether an action or behavior is harmful or beneficial to yourself; the other axis is based on whether an action or behavior is harmful or beneficial to others. These four sections, or zones, are as follows:

**Unfortunate zone**: The actions or behaviors benefit others and hurt yourself. These types of people are also called the helpless people, in the unfortunate or helpless zone.

**Bandit zone**: The actions or behaviors benefits yourself at the detriment of others. This is pure, ruthless greed. Think big tobacco denying they knew that cigarettes were addictive and harmful so as not to affect profits.

**Stupid zone**: The actions or behaviors not only hurt others, they hurt yourself, or at least you gain no benefit.

**Intelligent zone**: This is the win-win of them all, where the actions or behaviors benefits both you and others.

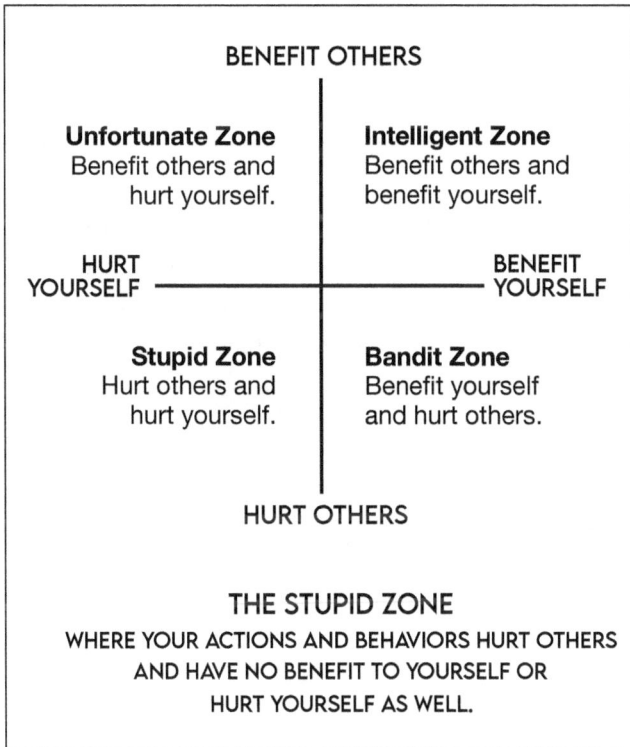

**BENEFIT OTHERS**

**Unfortunate Zone**
Benefit others and hurt yourself.

**Intelligent Zone**
Benefit others and benefit yourself.

**HURT YOURSELF** ———————— **BENEFIT YOURSELF**

**Stupid Zone**
Hurt others and hurt yourself.

**Bandit Zone**
Benefit yourself and hurt others.

**HURT OTHERS**

**THE STUPID ZONE**
WHERE YOUR ACTIONS AND BEHAVIORS HURT OTHERS AND HAVE NO BENEFIT TO YOURSELF OR HURT YOURSELF AS WELL.

Things to remember from Cipolla's hypothesis:

1. Non-stupid people are accountable. They take responsibility for their mistakes and owning them. When you blame others for your mistakes, you are demonstrating your lack of accountability, and possible lack of intelligence.
2. In conflict situations, intelligent people gather all relevant sources of information, including new and controversial information, to develop a well-informed opinion. Smart people are more open to listening to the opposing arguments and potentially reconsidering their own opinion. Stupid people tend to rant and rave they're right and the world is wrong.
3. Stupid people are more likely to react to confrontation with anger or aggression.
4. Smart people are empathetic and are more inclined to be helpful. Non-smart people are always looking to see what's in it for them.
5. Smart people are always trying to improve themselves. Non-smart people just think they are better than everyone else.[95]

> *Everybody is a genius. But if you judge a fish*
> *by its ability to climb a tree, it will live its*
> *whole life believing that it is stupid.*
> —ALBERT EINSTEIN

The human ability to work with our fellow humans has been the driving factor in our survival. Of course, from time to time we're looking out for ourselves and putting our needs first, but in general, if you work well with others, that could mean the most important signifier of intelligence. Cooperation brought us together to accomplish greatness and survive.

Of course, everyone is guilty of dipping into the Stupid Zone. But if the shoe is starting to fit pretty well, then you're not dipping into the Stupid Zone; you're living in it.

# THINK WEEK—IGNITING CURIOSITY

Somewhere among the cedar trees of the Pacific Northwest, there's a secluded cabin stocked with Diet Orange Crush and Diet Coke. Twice a year, it's inhabited by Bill Gates for a ritual known as "Think Week." Bill spends the week alone reading, sometimes eighteen hours at a stretch or well into the night. The purpose is for Gates to separate from everything and ponder the future of technology and how to make the world a better place.[96]

One of the biggest complaints about modern life is that information is coming at us with the force of a fire hose. It makes it so hard to clear the noise and think. Think Week is not about being Zen, but about being able to remove the constant chatter so we can go deeper into problems. It allows us time to figure things out away from the distractions and pace of our normal lives. Freeing thought allows our curiosity to bloom.

Curiosity is the desire to explore, to embrace complex, unfamiliar circumstances, and ambiguous events, to experience discovery, and most importantly, to feel the joy of it all. Even idle curiosity—wanting to know things for no specific reason—is a good thing. If it weren't for curiosity, we wouldn't be the advanced species on earth that we are.

Curiosity helped us to survive. We created new tools to help adapt to our continually changing environment. Everything around us started with the questions: What if? What if I could figure out how to do something? Our need to survive and search for ways to make our survival easier may be why our brains evolved to release the feel-good chemicals. When we encounter new and exciting things, it prompts the release of dopamine, increasing our motivation to learn and figure things out. It inspires our brain to both enjoy the process of learning and remember what we've learned.

Curiosity is a candle that needs to be lit. We need stimulation for the flame to ignite. There needs to be a spark. Some scientists consider curiosity an urge, like hunger or thirst, that needs to be satisfied. Is curiosity part of our nature, or does motivation spark it?

*I have no special talents. I am only passionately curious.*
−ALBERT EINSTEIN

Curiosity is the motivation to seek new and different knowledge. Making discoveries lights up our brain with the thrill of making an accomplishment. The littles things, like cooking a new recipe, fire up that reward center so that we're happy with ourselves. Satisfaction equates to happiness.

**The cure for boredom is curiosity.**
**There is no cure for curiosity.**
−DOROTHY PARKER, AMERICAN POET

Deep within us is the drive to create. What you create doesn't have to be big. Find something, anything, that inspires or motivates you, and use it. Fuel your sense of creativity. The key is to find joy and be inspired by the everyday world. When we do something we like, great or small, we can be in the moment and genuinely enjoy it. The little things can become big and fill you with a great deal of joy and happiness.

## MULTI-HYPHENATES ARE THE MOST NONBORING PEOPLE

Dr. Jared Diamond is a perfect example of a multi-hyphenate, a person with multiple accolades, interests, education, skills and expertise in multiple areas. Dr. Diamond is best known for his popular Pulitzer Prize-winning books, *Collapse, Guns, Germs, and Steel,* and most recently, *Upheaval,* among others. That makes him a hugely successful author, a significant feat in itself—but there's more. He has a Bachelor of Arts in anthropology and a PhD in physiology. He has extensively studied ornithology and ecology, specializing in New Guinea. He was a professor of physiology at UCLA medical school but now is a professor of geography at UCLA. How does it all fit into one head?

Thomas Edison, perhaps most famous for inventing the light bulb, held over one thousand patents. When he was visiting a friend, his friend asked him to sign the guest book. In the space marked, "Interested in," Thomas Edison wrote: "Everything."

Dr. Jared Diamond and Thomas Edison are extreme examples of multi-hyphenates. All of us have the curiosity within us to be multihyphenates and learn multiple skills. When you love the things you do, it's hard to see them as work.

*I never did a day's work in my life. It was all fun.*
—THOMAS EDISON

## WHY DO WE HAVE TO LEARN WHAT WE ALREADY KNOW?

Learning is the process of drawing connections between what's already known or understood and new information. It's the domino effect of bringing in prior knowledge to solve new problems. We make comparisons with new information and existing information stored in our brain. When the brain finds a useful match, it eliminates the old and rewires in the new. From the moment we're born, our brains are hardwired to learn. To learn is to acquire new knowledge, understand more about ideas, satisfy our sense of curiosity, and improve our efficiencies by figuring out new ways to do things.

There are several ways to improve your cognitive plasticity. You would think some ways have nothing to do with learning. For example, it appears calorie-restriction or fasting promotes neuron growth because the shift in metabolism causes the body to produce lower amounts of leptin, (the satiety hormone we talked about earlier), and the brain's neurons then produce more energy.

Travel creates a situation where the brain is exposed to new and complex environments, causing the brain to sprout dendrites—short-branched extensions of the brain's nerve cells along which the synapses are transmitted.

There's nothing like exercise to push fresh blood through the brain. Dancing, especially a free-style form of dance that doesn't retrace memorized steps, seems to have the most significant effect on warding off neurodegenerative diseases than any other type of brain-stimulating activity. Researchers found people who boogied down had the most considerable reduction—76 percent—as opposed to those who read, with a 35 percent reduction. Dancing "forces you to integrate several brain functions all at once—kinesthetic, rational, musical, and emotional"—which boosts your cognitive stimulation.[97]

Other ways to improve your brain plasticity include creative learning processes such as expanding your vocabulary, reading, learning to play a musical instrument, doing brain games, doing memory games or techniques, creating artwork, using your nondominant hand for simple tasks, and learning any new skills. The point is always, always, always keep learning.

Don't ever stop!

Learning and acquiring knowledge is a repetitive activity. Some people learn best through visual stimulation, while some are more auditory driven. For example, are you a webinar person or a podcast kind of learner? Absorbing information and storing knowledge, takes practice and repetition. It's not a one-time event for things to stick.

Making knowledge sticky requires the knowledge to be repeated, practiced, and honed. Hermann Ebbinghaus, of the Ebbinghaus forgetting curve, theorized that people forget about 50 to 80 percent of what they learned just days after learning it. The key to learning and retaining core content and critical points is repetition especially when repeated with consistent spaced out internals.

To test his hypothesis, Ebbinghaus developed a list of twenty-three hundred nonsense syllables like "zuc" and "qax." He then set out to remember sets of syllables and test different lengths and intervals for learning, noting the speed of learning and forgetting what he had learned. He then compared the curve of forgetting to the curve of memorizing more enjoyable groups of words.

Not surprisingly, it was easier to recall a lovely poem rather than a similar length of nonsense syllables. His conclusion: remembering meaningful things had more significance and was easier to recall than those nonsensical things. He also noted we start forgetting within the first hour, and after twenty-four hours, about two-thirds of anything learned is forgotten. This is why learning is challenging, but repetition will make it engrained.[98]

# THE KAIZEN WAY

*Kaizen* is the Sino-Japanese word for "improvement." The kaizen way is a belief that continuous, incremental improvements add up to the changes that make a difference over time. Three basic principles will help you improve your daily habits and productivity.[99]

1. Determine where you spend your time and energy.
2. What small, incremental steps can you make to be more productive with your time and energy?
3. Review what's working: What's getting in the way of progress, and what needs improvement?

One of the mistakes in self-improvement is we go after the big answers, but to get to the big answers, we have to get through all the little stuff. There are no short cuts. Small, daily habits are more important than the occasional big leap. It's the small daily steps that lead to the leaps and bounds. It's the small steps that make it all doable.

> *Life is made up of small pleasures. Happiness is made up of those tiny successes. The big ones come too infrequently. And if you don't collect all these tiny successes, the big ones don't really mean anything.*
> —NORMAN LEAR, TV PRODUCER

We'll buy into the promise of six-pack abs in thirty days. The big answer is getting ripped abs, but there's still the fact you have to do the work. The only way to get those six-pack abs is to do the exercise, diet, and work at it every day. The little decision of everyday habits, in every way, one by one, start to finish, one step at a time, is the way to achieve any goal. You don't get there without the small incremental daily decisions.

The kaizen way method can be used in your business or personal life. By breaking apart the process of anything you do, then putting it back together with as little wasted time or energy as possible, you'll see improvements in your life.

On the smallest scale, if you want to be more organized, you could start with a basic habit tool. Every night, take ten minutes to jot down three things you want to accomplish the next day. Over the weekend, take a half hour and jot down what you want to achieve in the coming week. At the new year, jot down your plan for the coming year. It's the small, incremental steps of awareness that will keep you on track to accomplish your goals.

# BEING CHECKED INTO PERFECTION

With the sounds of crickets and a distant train whistle, Corsicana, Texas, is the epitome of a small town. It's mostly known for the million-plus fruit cakes made at the Collins Street Bakery and as home to Navarro College, a two-year community college. The story of the Corsicana might have ended with that except for something else extraordinary, the Navarro College Cheer Team.

Under Head Coach Monica Aldama's direction, Navarro College Cheer Team has won fourteen NCA (National Cheer Association) National Championships and five NCA Grand National Championships since 2012 making their record untouchable and the absolute best of the best.[100]

There's the image of college cheerleaders standing on the sidelines encouraging the crowd to show support for the team. That's a very small part of the Navarro Cheer Team's activities. The majority is the brutal, daily practice to prepare for the NCA National Cheerleading Championship held in Daytona Beach, Florida, every April.

The entire year is spent practicing the routine for the two-minute and fifteen-second performance. One misstep in the performance, and your entire year and life of practice is done. Just to be on the team, many of these kids were training for years, some from the time they can walk. It takes so much to get to the level of a Navarro Cheer Team member, and it could take only a split-second in competition to screw it up.

Other collegiate team sports like basketball or football, you can turn pro. But there's no afterlife for collegiate cheer teams. There's no turning professional. It's not an Olympic sport. Cheerleading is not a career track that will lead to a job performing, like an ice skater might join the Ice Capades. After college, you're done. Your career is over.

That makes it all the more important to understand what goes into becoming one of the best for a cheer team. The unique stunts and aerial acrobatics require a level of athleticism not seen in any other sport. They're equal parts gymnast, aerial flyer, Cirque du Soleil performer, and dancer. Not only does each individual have a high skill set, but they also have to trust that their team members will do their parts. Their lives literally depend on it.

The two-minute and fifteen-second performance has a multitude of eye-popping stunts culminating in what's known as the pyramid—people stacked three up, balanced in formation. "Tumblers" have to do strings of flips, back handsprings, and other aerial acrobatics and make it look effortless. "Flyers" are the ones that get jettisoned into the air, spinning and flipping, peaking about two to three stories high. Then gravity pulls them back, and they land with an audible thud into the arms of the "bases," those who are there to catch them. One miscalculation, and you are bug splat on the floor.

> **The way that we prepare, you keep going until you get it right, and then you keep going until you can't get it wrong.**
> —MONICA ALDAMA, HEAD COACH, NAVARRO COLLEGE CHEER TEAM

There's no other sport like this where you have to deeply trust each other with your life. Each member of the team knows the others will be there, checked in, ready to protect you from a tragic fall. When you become that close, you become a family. The absolute essence of a family is you can trust the other will be there for you and protect you. That's the Navarro Cheer Team.[101]

Do it until you get it right, then keep going until you can't get it wrong, is a philosophy that can work with everything in your life. Whether it's your job, family life or your own personal goals. Practice does make it as perfect as possible.

*Practice does not make perfect.*
*Only perfect practice makes perfect.*
−VINCE LOMBARDI, AMERICAN FOOTBALL PLAYER

# TEN THOUSAND HOURS MAKES FOR A GOOD START

Malcolm Gladwell, in his book *Outliers*, popularized the concept of practicing for ten thousand hours to advance from a novice into a level of professional or mastery of a craft. The ten thousand hours might break down into about twenty hours per week for ten years. The ten-thousand-hours rule is popular, but is it all that simple? Recent science says it takes more than just putting in the hours.

*Luck is where opportunity meets preparation.*
−SENECA, ROMAN PHILOSOPHER

In a study, a group of researchers picked two sets of students who were studying the violin on a serious level. In the first group were students whose music professors thought they had star-worthy talents. Let's call this group the stars. They also put together another group: students who were serious about the violin, but not in the same league as the stars. We'll call this group the mediocres. Both groups, the stars and the mediocres, were asked to make detailed logs of their practice sessions.

Surprisingly, both groups practiced about fifty hours a week. There was no difference in devotion to time between those who were on their way to world-class—the stars—and the mediocres. Since the hours of practice were about the same, what was it that elevated the elite stars over the mediocres?

Two things were discovered.

First, the star group spent three times more time on practices that pushed themselves and stretched their abilities—the uncomfortable, difficult and purposeful practice. They were challenging themselves always and not just repeating what they already knew.

Second, the star players consolidated their practice session to two long uninterrupted sessions, one in the morning and one in the afternoon. In contrast, the mediocres scattered their times throughout the day. The stars put in longer, harder sessions, pushing their skills, but expressed being significantly more relaxed than the mediocres. The star players were able to put in the hard, uncomfortable work, then leave it behind and enjoy their leisure time. The mediocres did short sessions through-out the day, stopping and starting up again, maybe never really getting the momentum they needed to push themselves.

The stop-and-go of the mediocres never got them into the deep rhythm, the immersion of pushing themselves, and the intensity and focus the star players worked with.

The quantity of playing, as in the ten-thousand-hours rule, doesn't appear to be the winner here. It is not the quantity, but the quality and intensity of the practice.[102]

I know when it comes to the things I wanted to accomplish in my life, it was the focused session that paid off. To get to the hard work, you have to go through the easy stuff. Like fitness training or writing this book, I wouldn't have made the progress I made if I had not put in long, dedicated hard sessions for both.

In weight training, using low weights to do reps will undoubtedly help you gain a level of fitness. But if you want to increase strength and stamina, you have to push it with heavier weights and more reps to fatigue the muscles. You've got to feel you're going to break. The same as playing the violin—if you want to be better, you've got to push yourself past your comfort level. You have to push it to your limits and then some more.

With weights, many people do three sets of reps. The number of reps varies depending on what you are doing. In the first set of reps, the brain is just trying to connect to the muscles and the movements. It usually winds up being a little clumsy. Then you rest before the second set.

In the second set, the body and mind are more connected, the move-ments are cleaner and not as jerky. But it's the third set of reps where the body and mind have gone through the preliminary work and are fully in sync. The muscles are now fatigued, but you push anyway. That's where the magic happens. You've got to go through the process to get to the last few reps when your muscles are screaming stop, but you push it. That's the juice. That's where you build strength and stamina. Everything before those last harder-than-hell reps is mere preparation.

For me, writing was no different. If I tried to write for twenty minutes here and there throughout the day as I wavered between tasks, my writing would have suffered. Stopping and starting means your brain has to spend time shifting between tasks, recalling where you were, and figure out what to write next, causing you to spend so much time with recall and revisiting where you left off. It was the long, marathon stretches that got me deep into the zone of my thoughts and challenged me to write complete sections.

Like "Think Week" for Bill Gates, the brain needs to be pushed. It's as essential as physical exercise. The brain's plasticity, its ability to modify its connections and rewire itself, is the process of learning, and the brain never stops changing in response to learning. No matter what your age.

*We do not rise to the level of our expectations.*
*We fall to the level of our training.*
—ARCHILOCHUS, GREEK POET

# THE DECISION-MAKING PROCESS OF LOGIC

Logic may seem like a boring robotic subject, but the truth is no decision is made without it. We need a world ruled by logic; otherwise, everything goes willy-nilly and makes no sense, and we fall into conflict, arguing over who's right and who's wrong. For example, in 1893, Orlando Ferguson believed the Earth was flat, but through the science and logic he was proven wrong.

Emotions power us, and I'll get to the importance of emotions later, but for now, let's focus on how logic makes sense of it all. Arguments based in logic bring us together and provides a beautiful framework for people to find common ground in a disagreement.

In many ways, logic is the soul of our intellect.

Logic is our most basic thinking tool. Every day, we analyze choices and situations to come up with solutions. All critical thinking or logic requires us to use reasoning skills to study a problem objectively and make rational conclusions about how to proceed.

Aristotle, the Greek philosopher and father of reasoning, died in 322 BC. One of his most significant accomplishments was to transform the subject of logic by developing syllogism. A syllogism is a form of logic in which an argument is made up of three propositions. Two of these propositions set out a statement, and the third proposition forms a conclusion from the combination of those two statements.

1. Proposition one: If it walks like a duck.
2. Proposition two: And quacks like a duck.
3. Conclusion: It must be a duck.

Syllogism depends on a precise arrangement of terms. In Aristotle's argument, he made the following:

1. Proposition one: All men are mortal.
2. Proposition Two: Socrates, Plato, and Aristotle are men.
3. Conclusion: Therefore, Socrates, Plato, and Aristotle are mortal.

Even today, Aristotle's syllogistic logic holds up nicely as a useful tool for making logical decisions. Let's take the example of Bob asking Mary out on a date. Mary doesn't know Bob, but she saw Bob at a party last week. He seemed to be having a good time talking with mutual friends. And Bob is hot! Before Mary says yes, the most logical thing would be for her to ask around and find out more about Bob.

1. Bill thinks Bob's a dirtbag because he stole money out of his wallet.
2. Betty thinks Bob's a dirtbag because he got Barbara pregnant while dating Sue.
3. In conclusion, Bob's a dirtbag. Say no to Bob.

Thank you, Aristotle.

Aristotle's syllogistic rule was embraced by the philosophical world up until the nineteenth century, when a fellow by the name of George Boole came along.

George Boole was a self-taught mathematician and philosopher, and his crowning jewel was his revelations in logic. He established modern symbolic logic an algebra of logic, now called Boolean algebra. If you do anything on a computer, you're using his method of logic. His genius discovery is a form of algebra based on a binary system of TRUE or FALSE and assigned either a 1 or a 0, like binary codes on a computer.

Boolean logic expresses a value that can be either true or false. Boole used operators OR, AND, and NOT to compare values and return a true or false result.

AND is used to target a group.

All conditions must be met for the value to be true.

For example, anyone who likes *puppies* AND *kittens*.

OR is used when one of two or more conditions are met.

When they are then the value is true.

For example, anyone who likes *puppies* OR *kittens*.

NOT is used to exclude people from a target group through the use of the exclusion. For example, anyone who likes *puppies*, NOT *kittens*.

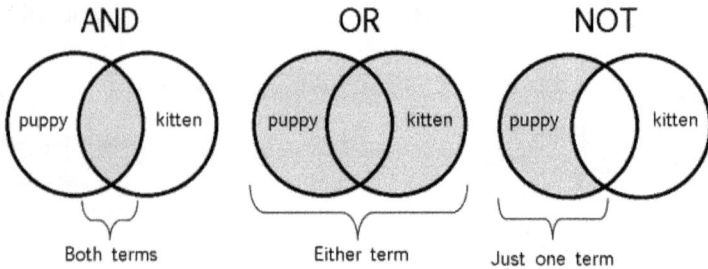

Boolean logic involves a series of statements, each of which must be true for the outcome to be true.

True or false, yes or no, rational or not—like little battles won, mini accomplishments, or mini discourse, logic is a small part of every decision we make. But could our decision-making process be that simple? How do we apply logic in our lives?

Sherlock Holmes, a fictional private detective created by Sir Arthur Conan Doyle, is known for his use of forensic science and logic to assist Scotland Yard in the 1880s.

*I never guess. It is a shocking habit—*
*destructive to the logical faculty.*
—SHERLOCK HOLMES

Dr. Spock was also a fictional character who was created for the sci-fi TV series *Star Trek*. He serves aboard the starship *Enterprise* as the science officer, with a personality built on his logical reasoning. Spock is half human and half Vulcan, a species known for their logic.

> **Logic is the beginning of wisdom ... not the end.**
> —DR. SPOCK

For these beloved characters, logic is an endearing personality trait. They systematically figure everything out, and we loved them for it. But these characters are fictional. As practical as it sounds, logic as a solitary tool for decision-making is rare for us mere mortals. We need more than spreadsheets and litmus tests, we need intuition.

Sometimes, we need to trust what's inside us—our gut.

## INTUITION—GOING WITH YOUR GUT

Steve Jobs called intuition, "more powerful than intellect." Intuition is elusive to define, but we all know what it is and how it feels, and we have all experienced it.

> **It's different from thinking, it's different from logic or analysis ... It's a knowing without knowing.**
> —SOPHY BURNHAM, AUTHOR, *THE ART OF INTUITION*

It's common to think our intuition arises organically, holistically, as a hunch or beacon of inner knowing to steer our decisions. But our intuition is our nonconscious thinking on autopilot. It may be defined as mental processing that works automatically with little analysis or information. With little critical thinking involved, our gut or intuition just knows. If something doesn't feel right, then something must be wrong. We may not know exactly what's wrong, but we just know something is wrong. Therefore, going with our gut instinct or intuition contributes highly to the decision-making process—maybe more than we know.

*Merriam-Webster* defines intuition as "quick and ready insight."

For example, we get clues from just looking at someone's face to know what they're feeling. Our bank of human emotions and past experiences bring us to an immediately judge whether this person is happy, sad, hurting, or upset.

Another example of autopilot intuition is highway hypnosis. This occurs when a driver has traveled miles without consciously thinking about the activity of driving the car. Our nonconscious thinking is safely driving the car while our consciousness is left for high-level thinking. Like what to say at the meeting you're about to attend, when to pick up the kids or that you need to add milk to the grocery list.

Our intuition can also lead us to make split-second decisions on complicated matters. Scientists have repeatedly demonstrated how what we know is stored in the brain without our conscious awareness. This bank of knowledge stored in the garage rafters of our brain can be brought to the surface in a flash.

In 1920, Albert Einstein said, "All great achievements of science must start from intuitive knowledge. At times, I feel certain I am right while not knowing the reason."

Malcolm Gladwell's book *Blink: The Power of Thinking Without Thinking*, highlights mental processing that works automatically, or our intuition. One example in the book highlights the Greek *kouros*, a dolomitic marble sculpture dating from the sixth century BC that was purchased by the J. Paul Getty Museum.

The art dealer had produced a string of legal documents proving the provenance. A geologist determined that the statue was covered in calcite, which dolomite can turn into only after hundreds of years. After months of investigation, the Getty concluded it was the real McCoy and bought it for ten million dollars. The documents were in order and the statue was covered with thousand-year-old dust; what other proof could there be? It must be authentic.

Not so fast.

Proud of the new purchase, the Getty displayed the piece and invited art historians to view the prized acquisition. One historian mentioned that, "it didn't look right." Another said her "instinctive sense" told her that something wasn't right. It was the head of the Acropolis Museum in Athens, George Despinis, who said he thought it was fake because when he saw it, he felt "intuitive repulsion."

There are fewer than two hundred similar kouros pieces left in existence, most are in bad condition or worse, in pieces. The one the Getty had purchased was near perfect. A second review of the documentation revealed some errors in postal dates and bank account numbers. It was soon discovered the kouros also resembled a forged one that came out of a workshop in Rome around 1980. And it turns out potato mold can age dolomite in only a few months.

The art historians used their life-time of stored knowledge, bridging the gap between conscious and nonconscious parts of the mind, and in an instant, they knew the statue was fake.[103]

> *We don't have to reject scientific logic ... in order to benefit from instinct. We can honor and call upon all of these tools, and we can seek balance. And by seeking this balance we will finally bring all of the resources of our brain into action.*
> — FRANCS CHOLLE, AUTHOR, THE INTUITIVE COMPASS

In an experiment, college students were shown a series of black-and-white images of dots that moved on half of a computer screen. The students were asked to report which way the dots were moving, right or left. When they answered, flashes of colors appeared on the other half of the screen. Hidden in some flashes of color were either positive images, like a puppy, or negative images, like a snake. These images were so fast they were imperceptible to the students except on the subliminal, unconscious level. The flashes were meant to stimulate the brain's process of intuition.

The results showed more accurate responses from the students who saw positive images in the flashes. They also responded quicker and felt more confident in their answers. This group's results have to do with our ability to take what the subconscious perceives and bring it to usefulness in the conscious brain when making decisions.[104]

Intuition heightens when you're more observant of your own mental and emotional processes. It's that moment when you just know. You understand what's in front of you completely without the need for detailed reasoning, bridging the gap between the conscious and the deeper subconscious part of the mind.

Some people trust their gut more than any other factor in making decisions because they've worked at it. Gut instinct, or intuition, involves the subconscious brain taking in the slightest details and feeding that information into the intuitive process of their conscious mind.

In the age of information overload—analysis paralysis—the intuition may sometimes get lost. It's important to pay attention to your gut feeling. Listen to the inner voice and ascribe value to the voice, the unconscious reasoning that we all have. Solitude, fewer distractions, and to unplugging might allow us to reconnect with ourselves and our intuition. Practicing mindfulness through meditation helps tap into our deepest creativity and connects us to our inner monologue.

We all receive messages in different ways. The key is being able to tap into them. Intuition doesn't replace logic; rather, reasoning and logic can be your checklist against what your intuition knows to be true. Logic and intuition are both parts of our innate knowing.

*Intuition comes very close to clairvoyance; it appears to be the extrasensory perception of reality.*

—ALEXIS CARREL, NOBEL PRIZE IN PHYSIOLOGY

## PASSION AND PURPOSE

Where's the passion in the decision-making?

Our emotions compel us into action and influence all our decisions, both large and small. Our emotions can be fleeting and short-lived or complex, deep, and long term. Like our shadow on a sunny day, our emotions cling to us, following us around, never leaving our side. Every decision we make has a shadow of emotions tied to it.

Passion and the discovery of your innate talents are born from trying new things. You will never know what you love until you try it. Passion is a natural human fuel that inspires us into action. It's a form of energy that can improve focus and self-determination, putting you into a sense of flow. Work with passion becomes deeply satisfying.

It's said money often follows your passion. Sometimes that's true, but there's more than money involved in cultivating your passions or talents: it's about living a life with purpose.

Talent, aptitude, and intelligence are very democratic. You can't buy them. Opportunity may not be so democratic, but that can't stop you from pursuing your purpose and passions. There are very successful, talented people who don't have an advanced or college degrees. Ellen

DeGeneres, Ted Turner, Russell Simmons, and my personal favorite, Steve Jobs, were driven by their talents and passions. They never earned advanced degrees; they saw an opportunity and just went for what made them happy.

> *People often remark that I'm pretty lucky. Luck is*
> *only important in so far as getting the chance to*
> *sell yourself at the right moment. After that, you've*
> *got to have talent and know how to use it.*
> —FRANK SINATRA, SINGER

To discover what you want to do, begin with the end in mind. We have no control over who gave us our beginnings and our genetics. We were born with different strengths and weaknesses, into different environments, and with different parents, teachers, and mentors guiding us. We're not all born superathletes like LeBron James, or with the vocal strengths of Lady Gaga.

> *Following your genuine intellectual curiosity is*
> *better than following whatever makes money. The*
> *internet has massively broadened the space of*
> *possible careers. Most people don't understand this.*
> —NAVAL RAVIKANT, ANGELLIST, STARTUP INVESTOR

Information flows freely. You can learn anything you want. The Internet, books, documentaries, and libraries make information available to everyone. With access to a computer and the Internet, your circumstances no longer limit your availability to knowledge. All the answers are out there, just waiting for you to find them and use them in your own life.

It takes hard work, the courage to do it, and a deep sense of curiosity. Intelligence comes in many forms. You can develop practical knowledge, be creative or analytical or a mix of them all. But there is also emotional intelligence which has to do with our self-esteem, self-awareness, motivation, empathy and how we deal with others. In the next chapter, we will look at tactics to find your own mojo and what true success really means.

---

## CHAPTER SUMMARY

☑ Approach knowledge with curiosity, enthusiasm, and passion.

☑ Emotions are neither good nor bad. Like the weather, they come and go. Anger fades. Love can be timeless.

☑ Use logic and intuition to make your decisions.

☑ Keep learning and discovering.

☑ Mistakes happen. Learn from them.

---

## CHAPTER THIRTEEN

# Esteem

*Fear of failure is caused by lack of self-esteem and confidence. Dealing with fear is the key to super success.*

— DAN PEÑA, FOUNDER, QLA (QUANTUM LEAP ADVANTAGE)

## ARE YOU SMACK-TALKING YOURSELF?

We are often far harder on ourselves than others would be. Why?

Our ancestral brain needed us to keep the tribe alive for the human race to survive. To accommodate the importance of the tribe, we were hardwired to care for others. Our brain saw someone in distress, and we jumped into action to help. Today's world is no different. We do the same. We care for our friends. We reach out to them in difficult times. But do we treat ourselves as well as we treat a friend?

The answer comes down to neuroscience—the chemicals rolling around in our brain—and how the brain is wired. Our brains are wired to care about the well-being of others, our friends, and our tribe, but that same system doesn't seem to kick in when we're berating and beating ourselves up over our own mistakes and shortcomings.

We have to go back to our fight-or-flight mode to learn why. Kristin Neff,

PhD, a professor at the University of Texas at Austin, helps us understand how fight or flight contributes to us downplaying self-compassion:

*When a friend fails, you don't feel threatened. You can easily access a part of your physiology: the caregiving system. As mammals, we all have part of ourselves that is devoted to caregiving for a friend in need. But when I'm threatened, my natural response is a fight, flight, or freeze. Now, of course, that system developed in order to protect our bodily self, but the problem is that when we fail, our self-concept gets threatened, and our body reacts exactly the same way. When we feel threatened, we can't access the caregiving system. Our most immediate and strongest reaction is this fight-or-flight response. We fight the problem — which is ourselves. We attack ourselves, we judge ourselves, or we feel really isolated. In a way, I think that's the reason it's so much easier to be kind to others than ourselves, because we aren't threatened by others' problems. We are being hard on ourselves, and we're tapping into the reptilian brain as opposed to the more mature caregiving area.[105]*

Self-compassion means treating yourself as you would a close friend. When you're troubled or full of self-doubts, and self-criticism, ask yourself, What would I say to a friend in a similar situation? Chances are it would be solid, heartfelt advice. We all need love and encouragement, advice, and support from each other, and the world needs you to do the same for yourself.

# IS THE GLASS HALF EMPTY OR HALF FULL?

We're not meant to be pessimists or succumb to helplessness—it's not the dominant behavior in our nature. Otherwise, we never would have survived. It's a learned behavior, and if it's learned, then it can be unlearned.

In his TED Talk, Dr. Guy Winch explains how perceived failure is as painful as our own failure. Meaning when we see failure in others, we sometimes adopt their feelings of the experience as our own. We can feel the joy of others as well as we can feel others' failures.

In his presentation, he talks about visiting a day-care facility where three toddlers were playing with toy pop-up boxes. If you pushed the right button on the toy box, a doggie would pop up. One child tried, kept pushing and pulling the wrong buttons to get the doggie to pop up. After a while she just gave up, with her lower lip trembling in defeat. The second toddler saw this and was so heartbroken at the first toddler's failure that the second toddler burst into tears without ever touching the toy. The third toddler kept trying until she pushed the right button; the doggie popped up, and she squealed with delight.

All three toddlers had the same toys but all very different reactions to failure. The first two could have kept going and were perfectly capable of eventually getting the toy doggie to pop up, but their minds chose to accept defeat and become helpless.

The feeling of helplessness comes when someone experiences repeated adverse situations and becomes unable or unwilling to avoid or change the situation. For example, cases of mental or physical abuse or repeated failures can trigger helplessness. Their brain has trained them to believe they have no control, so they give up or don't even try, as in the case of the first two toddlers.

We've all felt defeat at some point or another. The possibility of failing is part of attempting new things. However, when we fill our minds with limiting beliefs, we give into failure before even trying. This dangerously affects our motivation, and our overall productivity may needlessly suffer.

Learned helplessness is mostly unconscious. Whenever we experience feelings of negativity, the brain screams we shouldn't do what we're doing—fear of failure and rejection pops up. With enough of these instances, the brain experiences negative conditioned learning.

As adults, we encounter frustrations and setbacks. If your mind defaults to failure, we'll feel the needless sense of helplessness. So often we stop too soon, or we don't bother trying at all.[106]

If a behavior is reinforced or rewarded, we're more likely to repeat that behavior. Consequently, if we experience adverse outcomes or are punished, we're more likely to avoid that behavior in the future. Awareness of why you recoil, feel helpless, or have a defeatist attitude will help you overcome it and unlearn this association.

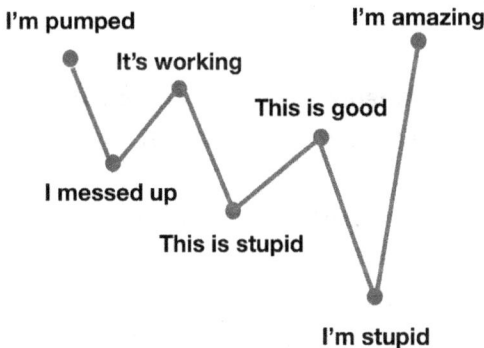

**I'm pumped**     **I'm amazing**
**It's working**
**This is good**
**I messed up**
**This is stupid**
**I'm stupid**

Exchange pessimistic behavior and tendencies for optimistic ones. Change the belief that failure is beyond your control by exploring the origins of your learned helplessness. Develop ways to decrease those feelings by identifying thoughts, behaviors, and actions that reinforce learned helplessness. Ask yourself, What thoughts do not serve me? Replace those thoughts and behaviors with positive ones that improve your self-esteem. Set realistic goals and ways to accomplish them.

*Success has been defined as the ability to go from failure to failure without losing enthusiasm.*
—DAVID GUY POWERS, AUTHOR

# FINDING YOUR MOJO

To start changing your limiting beliefs and boost your self-esteem, you first got to get your mojo on. Only then can you share your power with the world. Mojo is defined as good luck, charm or skill that seems to come from something magical or supernatural. Mojo is confidence on steroids.

Like the chrysalis turning into the butterfly, we grow and change. We have to; it's part of our nature. We want to make it to the other side, from struggle and discontent, to peace and contentment. The grass seems greener on the other side, but any grass will be greener where you water it. It's not about geography—it's about watering the grass right under your feet.

> ### *Wherever you go, there you are.*
> —JON KABAT-ZINN, UMASS CENTER FOR MINDFULNESS

Problems follow you everywhere you go. If you haven't made peace with yourself for things you've done in the past, you will be dealing with that baggage forever. If you're habitually late, moving closer to your office won't work. Your habits follow you. Change the pattern, not the location.

No amount of guilt can change the past, and no amount of worrying can change the future. Focus on today. Focus on the present and what can be done.

> ### **Do not regret past mistakes. All decisions, good and bad, led you to where you are today. (Disregard this if you're in prison.)**
> —ANONYMOUS

Fear holds us back. It's a rope tethering us to our past experiences or our future negative expectations, but it's a rope that can be severed.

Break it to move on and become the person you need to be, for yourself and the world.

There's one surefire way to jump-start your mojo, and that's to face your fears. It takes courage and the ability to do what scares the hell out of you.

No matter what mistakes you've made in the past, to get your mojo back, face a fear—any fear—and believe in yourself again. Believe you have what it takes to do anything you set your mind to do. It's life, baby, and that means challenges. Life is difficult. Doing your best is the best you can do.

*Courage is being scared to death, but saddling up anyway.*
—JOHN WAYNE

# LIFE-CHALLENGING EVENT NUMBER FOUR

Into the ocean I go, to lose my mind and find my soul.

As I have mentioned, I'm a surfer. When I say that, you might picture a tan, bikini-clad chick, riding the face of a wave like nothing else matters, then finishing with an air fist bump.

That's not me.

I surf off the coast of Los Angeles. Since the water there is pretty cold, I'm clad in a full-body wetsuit. The wetsuit is a dirty faded black with green chest stripes. For sun protection, I smear a heavy coat of zinc oxide sunscreen on my face and hands, making me look like I'm covered in ash. It's not a pretty picture. There's no tanned body or bikini under all that.

Surfing in Los Angeles takes a lot of work. You've got to really want it and there are at least a dozen reasons to chuck it all and go do yoga instead.

First, it takes a lot of gear and paraphernalia. There are wetsuits, surf-boards, surfboard racks on your car, sunblock, wax, leashes for the board, board bags, and you need water to rinse off with after, along with a mountain more of gear. Forget about keeping your car clean. The interior of your car winds up smelling like the sweaty ocean—in a bad way, the leather seats are scarred by the salt, and there's sand embedded in everything.

The beach where I surf is right on Pacific Coast Highway, with four lanes of traffic whizzing by. It's not the tropical palm-strewn beach most people dream about. To get down to the water, you have to maneuver around some big rocky boulders. On days when the surf is fast and rough, one misstep and the waves will pound you on those rocks like bug splat on a windshield.

The cardinal rule is never surf alone, so I do have a surf buddy who's as up for the torture as I am. When everything is coordinated: I find myself standing on Pacific Coast Highway. As four lanes of traffic meander by, I contort my body into a tight, rubberized neoprene wetsuit. There's no way to do that gracefully. My only hope is my wriggling might provide comedic fodder for those driving by.

Surfing is not for the faint of heart. It's physically challenging, and there's no way to make it easier. You're awkwardly laying prone, chest-high on a surfboard, paddling as hard as you can to get up and over oncoming waves. The waves smash you in the face like someone tossing a bucket of ice water at your head and, consequently, up your sinuses. The after-math is days of sore muscles and dripping sinuses. You've just got to be up for that.

Worst of all, the ocean takes no prisoners. It's a do-or-you-die situation. The ocean is not predictable. The waves change all the time. There's no sport like it—in tennis, golf, football, even skiing, the court or course is stable. Unlike the constant moving of the ocean.

You can't turn your back on the ocean for a second. Rogue waves come up all the time. Being in the wrong place when a rogue wave pops up is like turning to see the garage door about to come down on your head. It's a big, cavernous, dark monster about to swallow you alive. Then it does, and you find yourself being tossed and pulled, like a rag doll through the washing machine spin cycle of a wave. After holding your breath for what seems an eternity, you get spit out the backside, find a break in the waves to surface and suck in a quick breath.

The ocean demands your attention.

Some days I am fired up. I can't wait to get in the water, whether the waves are happening curls of perfection or crappy beach crashers. I just want to go out.

Other days I stand on the shore, looking out, and want to cry. My desire to cry has nothing to do with surf conditions; it's all in my head. I'll try to explain, but you won't truly understand until you skinny into a wetsuit and get your butt out in the unruly ocean.

The ocean has a soul. When you leave terra firma and paddle out into this amniotic fluid, your relationship with the world changes. You're no longer a part of the earth. You're disconnected from all that you've known.

You're free.

What I'm about to tell you is the opposite of being free, though.

I almost drowned as a kid.

I was at the Lake of the Ozarks standing at the end of a dock when I saw a boat towing a water-skier coming towards me. As I raised my hand to wave, the skier dumped and flung the tow rope. The rope accidentally wrapped around my arm, jerking me off the dock and into the water.

The rope, still twined around my arm, pulled me down to the depths of the lake, burning and dislocating my arm until it finally released.

I was lodged under a bunch of trees that had been sunk in the lake to attract fish for easier catching. I remember looking up and seeing the blackness tighten around me. The blotch of light above me seemed so far away. I was too stunned to move, and all went black.

Neither the skier nor the driver of the boat saw me standing on the dock. No one saw me go in except my dad, who was standing on a road up away from the lake. By a miracle, he made it in time to dive in and pull me out.

After that experience, I was terrified of water. I would panic and even pass out when I tried to swim in lakes or the ocean. The emotional anxiety seemed to sweep over me even though I knew in my heart I was safe. It was overwhelming, paralyzing fear.

The first time I attempted surfing, I was terrified.

It was in Hawaii. My stepson had arranged surf lessons for the family. We'd been going to Hawaii for years, and I always passed on the surf lesson portion of the trip, but this time it was different. I was tired of being paralyzed. Just looking at the ocean sometimes made me slip back into that deep black hole. This time, I was ready. I was doing this whatever the outcome.

I sobbed as I explained to the surf instructor my fears. He was reassuring and explained he would tow me out past the waves. That he would stay with me. Not to worry; he would take care of me.

I was terrified the whole way out. I wanted to walk on water back to shore. I clung to the top of my surfboard like a rat on a sinking ship.

He told me he was going to line up my surfboard with a wave and push me into it. He said the surfboard was big and stable, and not to worry, that I could do it. Then he pushed the board and yelled, "Stand up! Do it! Stand up!" And I did. I stood up.

Like hundreds of butterflies floating off my body, the weight of anxiety lifted away. I felt born again, baptized by an ocean wave into freedom from fear. It was an epiphany. I stood on the board and rode the wave. I was done with my fear of water. For the first time, I cried not because I was afraid but because I was free. The water was now my friend.

For me, the ocean is a place you go to find yourself. To discover the deepest part of yourself that needs to be set free. I still can't describe what goes on inside my head. I know I'm a better person for it. The ocean is a place where I work things out. There's a solitude like none other. You're alone out there, as apart from it all as you could be, just sitting on a surfboard with yourself. It's only sky above and the depth of the ocean below. You're so disconnected from the material world—you become more of you.

Fear in all its forms and for all its reasons is crippling. What's it going to take to realize it's a rope holding you down? We deal with our anxiety and fear in different ways. I feel free in the ocean. I smile. Sometimes I do cry, but it's for how happy I am, and I don't need to go in the ocean to know that.

I hope you find your ocean and free yourself from whatever fear is holding you down.

A few things to remember:

1. Your goal is not to be better than anyone else. It's to be better than you used to be.
2. If it doesn't challenge you, it won't change you.
3. Your life doesn't get better by chance. Change it yourself. Tap into that part of yourself that connects you to your higher power, to the universe, and to your own joy. Find your ocean and dive in.

## REBOOTING YOUR MOJO

My friend, Linda, is a journal-writing commando. At her home, there are hundreds of used journals stacked like paper pancakes. She has even more unused ones, waiting their turn for her to write, color, paste, and fill the empty parts with whatever seeps out from her. The abyss of white pages becomes soaked in her thoughts, dreams, prayers, aspirations, goals, bitch sessions, whining, and wailing. She might as well slice open an artery and let the blood flow out onto the page. It could not be more personal.

I once asked what she did with all of them. Did she go back and reread them? I got a "sometimes" kind of response and knew then they were not created as reference material; they are her emotional dumpsters. They're an official record of what she needs to get out and be done with—a mental, emotional boneyard.

Journaling is a beautiful way to get the brain poo out of the head. It's a way to free yourself of the negativity, sorrow, and pain and to record the joys of happy days. The art of journaling can be an echo of your thoughts and experiences. Getting it all out of the head allows your mind, spirit, and consciousness collectively to work in harmony, creating a void for whatever needs to come in.

It's a way of letting go so more of all the good stuff can come in—life, love, intuition and creativity.

## MOTTO MOJO

Years ago, American Express produced a series of commercials. It was called "My Project" and featuring celebrities making personal statements. For Oscar-winning director Martin Scorsese, it was, "To tell unforgettable stories." For Jim Henson, creator of the Muppets, it was, "To use laughter to help children learn." And for Ellen DeGeneres, talk-show host extraordinaire, it was, "To encourage people to dance to their own tune."

Around the same time, I went to a presentation by Dr. Robert Maurer. He explained the concept of the kaizen way and how taking small steps, one at a time, will change your life. His lecture made sense to me—small steps will lead to change and ultimately accomplish your goal, or set you on another path that makes more sense. In his lecture, he showed a lot of thought-provoking slides and graphs and some fantastic video clips. One video segment, in particular, struck a chord in me.

In 1950, Mother Teresa received permission from the Holy See to start her order, the Missionaries of Charity, whose mission was to love and care for those people nobody wanted. She cared for the sick and dying, including thousands of lepers. In 1979, she was awarded the Nobel Peace Prize. In her acceptance speech, her simple message crystallized her belief that "the poor must know that we love them." The video segment Dr. Maurer featured was of this tiny little woman moving about the sick and tending to their needs. She was filling a pot with water as she said in the voiceover, "Whatever you do, do with love."

How wonderful—do what you do with love. Do it with love. It rang over and over in my head, and the simplicity, strength, and beauty of this small sentence still brings a release and breeze of freshness to my psyche every time I recall it.

The concept of a personal life motto began to brew.

We all have goals. You want to become a lawyer, then get your under-graduate degree with grades good enough to get into a law school, put in the work, graduate, pass the bar, and bam—you're an attorney. Woo hoo! Goals are easy set, but tougher to accomplish. Goals are reached at a point in the future, and take some time to accomplish. During that time, you make changes, sometimes many changes. For example, if you want to quit smoking, lose weight, get a Ph.D., or learn digital photography—it all takes time and application of your energies to attain your goals.

A personal life motto is not a goal but a state of being. It sticks to you, haunts you to snap to and be a certain way, act a certain way, and it imparts a confident presence. Like a dog on a leash, it follows you wherever you go.

Mother Teresa: all she did, she did with love.

A personal life motto is one unique and differentiating phrase that sets your cosmic butt into action on your mission in this world. After I began thinking about my motto, I wondered, Did I have a cosmic quest, my yellow brick road to take me to the wizard? Maybe. But nothing came to me.

Bill Gates is known to be a walker, claiming it helps him reflect on thoughts and ideas, and to figure things out. I get that and use hiking to sometimes sort out my thoughts.

Living in Los Angeles, there's the Santa Monica Mountains right in your backyard. My favorite hike is a grueling six-miles through a remote part of a beautiful canyon. It's an uphill butt-buster. I like early mornings and I prefer the solitude of going alone.

The solitude lets my brain filter through the list of things to do, email messages to send, phone calls to make, car repairs, pick-ups, drop-offs, lions, and tigers, and bears, oh my!

But at some point, my brain becomes empty. My body hits a rhythm. My list of things to do becomes a whiteboard erased clean. I'm in sync with the trail, and my mind is a blank canvas. It's when the brain is empty, is when you can fill it with inspiration.

On this particular hike, I thought, What could I do for the world? Like the American Express ad campaign, what could be my life motto? It was a beautiful morning with soft shadows across the hillside. It made me happy and I raised my arms over my head and stretched my face towards the heat of the early morning sun. I thought, I am here in this world, and I have something to contribute. What resonated through my core was that I just wanted to help good people do good things. Maybe that could be my life motto—to help good people do good things. That felt right. I took a deep breath, turned, and walked on.

The meaning of my life motto is simple. I don't expect to do any great thing myself. I'm not Mother Teresa. I genuinely thought about what I could contribute to the world and kept coming up blank. I've seen dedicated people push the proverbial boulder up the hill just by their sheer determination. These are good people doing good things, and I realized I was best serving and helping them. I didn't need my own bolder. I needed them.

> *We are slowed-down sound, and light waves, a walking bundle of frequencies, turned into the cosmos. We are souls dressed up in sacred biochemical garments, and our bodies are the instruments through which our souls play their music.*
>
> —ALBERT EINSTEIN

## IT TAKES A VILLAGE

As a fifteen-year old boy, Arnold Schwarzenegger saw a magazine with Reg Park on the cover. Reg Park won the bodybuilding contest Mr. Universe, and went on to play Hercules in a chain of *Hercules* movies. Arnold was so inspired he took up weightlifting, and the rest is history. But what if he had never seen that magazine? We don't get anywhere alone. We receive our cues from all kinds of inspiration, but we still have to take actions ourselves. Or as motivational speaker Tony Robbins exclaims, "Take *massive* action!"

Arnold Schwarzenegger, born in 1947, grew up in Austria in a house without plumbing. At age twenty-one, speaking little English and with only a gym bag, he came to the United States. Within just a few years, he captured his first Mr. Olympia bodybuilding title. Arnold is an actor, filmmaker, an astute businessman, a real estate investor, an author, a former Mr. Universe, a seven-time Mr. Olympia winner, and a former governor of California. But he'll tell you straight out he's not a self-made man.

We don't get anywhere alone.

He was motivated and driven, but he'll admit it's the people in his life that fueled his dreams and made them happen. He credits his life to the support of parents, coaches, and teachers. It was all the people along the way, from the kind soul who let him sleep on a couch in the back of the gym, to the over four million people who voted him into the governorship. So many people gave him a little bit of help.

We need help. It's virtually impossible to go it alone. When it comes to your accomplishments, you're most likely there because of the help people gave you along the way. Motivation may only come from within, but it still takes a village to make it all work together. You won't get to where you want to be alone—so find your village.

## THE TRUE MEASURE OF SUCCESS

Quite often, success is related to achieving specific goals or accomplishments. Short-term goals are usually based on specific outcomes, like stepping stones in life—you complete one and move onto the next. Reaching these goals, like losing weight, learning to cook or learning a new language, all are related to learning a new skill. But the really good stuff happens when you think about your long-term life goals.

*Success is a peace of mind, which is a direct result of self-satisfaction in knowing you made the effort to do your best, to become the best that you are capable of becoming.*
—JOHN WOODEN, UCLA BASKETBALL COACH

Success is more than achieving wealth or fame. Being wealthy or famous does not guarantee happiness. Don't get me wrong—if you're having a horrible day, it's certainly more appealing to have a melt-down cry-fest in your Mercedes-Benz than sitting in your broken-down, beat-up clunker. Having beautiful things is nice, but money and fame don't feed the spark that makes us human.

What you do professionally to earn a living is not what defines you as a successful, productive member of society. We are all interdependent on everyone being and doing their best.

*A society grows great when old men plant trees in whose shade they know they shall never sit.*
—GREEK PROVERB

Success is not just one thing. You need skills, passion, determination, and the discipline to keep at it. And finally, you need luck. Luck to put you in the right place at the right time. Your success as a person starts with how you treat yourself. It doesn't matter what you do but how you do it, and how you do it is a direct result of your vision of self-worth and self-esteem. If you're doing your best, it trickles down and outward. Success leaves traces of our humanity. Success is not what you do—it's what you leave behind.

You're going to die. That's a fact. But your work lives on and makes your life memorable. In the end, your sole purpose in this universe is to add a little joy and make the world better.

*Do your little bit of good where you are; it's those little bits of good put together that overwhelm the world.*

—DESMOND TUTU, THEOLOGIAN

## SOMETIMES THE UNIVERSE SHOWS YOU THE WAY

January 2013. It had been years in the planning, but today was the day the doors opened for the Boys & Girls Club of Mar Vista Gardens at the Jack and Cindy Jones Youth Center.

My husband, Jack, had been working on this project for years. His idea was to do something significant for children. He thought the best organization to partner with would be the Boys & Girls Clubs of America, a non-profit institution that provides after-school programming for kids in kindergarten through high school. The Housing Authority of the City of Los Angeles (HACLA) had underused parks and recreation buildings that they would donate for use. It was a trifecta of good: a city-owned property, a nationally recognized nonprofit dedicated to kids, and a philanthropist all coming together to do one beautiful thing for children.

One saying kept rolling around in my head: children make up about 25 percent of the population, but they are 100 percent of our future. Wow, that sold me. I wanted to impact the future of kids, so my husband and I were all in.

Over the years since the grand opening, there have been gala dinners to honor us, news coverage, and accolades from every city, state, and government office. Senators, governors, members of Congress have shaken our hands and thanked us for our generosity. Magazine articles have been written about it, and thousands of people know who we are and what we've done.

All very nice, but I want to take you back to the day we first opened the facility.

We had decided a soft opening was best as we were working on plans to renovate and expand the facility. Once the plans were ready, we would close the building and set up double-wide trailers on the lawn area to accommodate the kids' programs. We thought a more appropriate time to do a big grand opening event would be after the renovation was complete. In the meantime, we wanted the kids to have a safe place to just be kids and get involved.

But something else happened that January afternoon. Something that took my breath away.

The doors opened at 3:00 p.m., and about thirty kids funneled in and were herded outside to the bleachers by the baseball diamond for the obligatory photo op. They all sat there excited and full of smiles as the club's new director went over the announcements.

"This is Jack and Cindy Jones. Their generosity funded the club." Blah, blah, blah.

Sitting a few rows ahead of us in the bleachers, one kid kept turning around to look at us. He was a big, kind of awkward, young African American boy dressed in an oversized T-shirt and silky basketball shorts. He stood out because of his size. He towered over all the other kids. I kept thinking, Why's this kid keep looking at us?

Photo op complete, a round of applause, and the kids were set free to enjoy the club.

Jack and I meandered toward the parking lot, stopping to thank the director and other staff members. We thanked the director for her kind words about us. Blah, blah, blah, dedication, enthusiasm and other stuff.

That's when I felt a tap on my shoulder.

It was the big, awkward kid. Huh?

He stuck out his hand and said, "I want to thank you for what you have done."

I lost it.

My eyes welling with tears, I realized what we had done was so much bigger than anything I could have ever imagined. One awkward kid wanting to shake my hand, was more important to me than any other accolade I could ever receive.

Today, there are over six hundred kids at the club. I have met and been involved with several of them. I have seen them grow from little snippets into people towering over me. I've witnessed them grow in so many other ways, too. Nothing else I've done has brought me so much happiness. More importantly, it has brought so much joy into the world.

It has put me outside of myself, on the other side of somewhere else.

> **What we have done for ourselves alone, dies with us; What we have done for others and the world, remains and is immortal.**
> —ALBERT PIKE, AMERICAN AUTHOR

## CHAPTER SUMMARY

☑ Keep learning.

☑ Dedicate 15 minutes to a troublesome task and see where it takes you.

☑ The things that define you are your patience when you have nothing, and your attitude when you have everything.

☑ Whatever you do, do it with love.

☑ Plant the seeds of ideas, good works and love. Water your garden. Help it grow. Repeat often.

☑ Striving for success without action behind it, is like trying to harvest where you haven't planted seeds.

☑ Success is how much good you can send into the world.

# Conclusion

## THE DECISIVE MOMENT

Henri Cartier-Bresson pioneered street photography using what he called the "decisive moment." He was a painter, but was inspired by photographs, so he took up photography in the 1930s and acquired a Leica camera with a 50-millimeter lens. This small camera allowed him to move freely through crowds. People change when they see a camera pointed at them, but Cartier-Bresson wanted to capture candid moments of real life, so he painted all the shiny parts of the camera black to make it as inconspicuous as possible.

"I suddenly understood that a photograph could fix eternity in an instant."

Cartier-Bresson's term "decisive moment," referred to capturing an event in its candid splendor, where the very essence of what is happening is ephemeral and spontaneous but captured forever in the photographic image.[107]

Why is this concept important?

Today is today, not tomorrow. Like the decisive moment, this moment is now, then gone forever. Did you use it wisely? When do you want your life to have true, deep purpose and love?

The road of life is paved with flat squirrels who couldn't decide. This is your decisive moment. Someday is today.

## GETTING IN THE *UN*COMFORT ZONE

The term *comfort zone* originally referred to a temperature zone of between 67 and 78 degrees where most of us are comfortable and feel neither hot nor cold.

Psychologically speaking, the comfort zone, as defined by Lifehacker, is a "behavioral space where your activities and behaviors fit a routine and pattern that minimizes stress and risk." The operative words here are *stress* and *risk* are *minimized*.

Safe, but is that how you want your life to go? Safe? Where's the adventure?

Within that zone, there is familiarity, certainty, and a sense of predict-ability in our routines. Outside is uncertainty, new stuff, possibly stuff we don't like, risk, and maybe even anxiety or stress. It can be scary to venture out of the comfort zone.

In the comfort zone, we've built preferences, like which restaurants we like, TV shows we want to watch, clothing brands, what friends to hang with, and whether to eat Doritos Jacked Ranch Dipped Hot Wings chips, or plain potato chips. We're comfortable in our comfort zone, where we've built our routines and systems to keep stress and anxiety at a minimum. Our comfort zone is great to have, and a won-derful support to fall back into when the world is too stressful. We've spent a lot of time building our comfort zone, so why would we ever think about leaving it?

When it comes to growth, the universal factor is we need to step out of our comfort zone and challenge ourselves. Growth comes only through challenges and trying new things. Anxiety and stress sometimes get a bad rap. A little anxiety or stress is a sign of anticipation—not always a bad thing. It's a sign of starting a new adventure too. Anxiety has the same symptoms as excitement, depending on how you look at it. For example, if you're anxious about giving a speech, maybe you can look at it as you're excited to give the speech. Similar feelings with different meanings.

Trying new things, learning new skills or even putting yourself in new environments can make you more creative. New things challenge our brains and lead to a rewiring of the brain's structure. New stuff means building new brain connections. It can be learning new skills, dancing a new step, meeting new people, doing activities that incorporate brain stimulations, attending a social engagement, participating in sports, or other physical activities—all these boost thinking skills and the brain's neuroplasticity.

> *In an increasingly competitive, cautious and accelerated world, those who are willing to take risks, step out of their comfort zone and into the discomfort of uncertainty will be those who will reap the biggest rewards.*
>
> —MAGGIE WARRELL, AUTHOR

Sometimes we feel pulled toward new and interesting people, things or events. We're curious about new concepts and want to learn more—meet new people, explore new cities, or see new things. We're drawn out of ourselves and into the unknown. The adventure into the unknown to see, be open to amazement, and learn.

Sometimes the pull just isn't there. Then, you need to take a leap out of your comfort zone. Like a baby bird looking down from the nest, open your wings into the abyss of the unknown, discover your innate talent—and fly.

Whether you're pulled by your own curiosity or take a leap of faith, put venturing into the *un*comfort zone on the list of things to do.

## THE BIG WRAP-UP

I will leave you with two very large decisions.

First: Your mind will not flourish without the health of your body. You simply must put your body first. The healthier the tree, the better the fruit. For yourself and for everyone in your life, you must put your body first. I can't say it enough.

> *The mind's first step to self-awareness*
> *must be through the body.*
> —GEORGE A. SHEEHAN, PHYSICIAN AND ATHLETE

Second: What goes on in the head, whatever you think, you will be. The neurochemical soup that's swimming around in your brain is all the emotions and intellectual stuff that make up the best part of being human. Your emotional health is as important as your physical health.

> *Whatever you think that you will be. If you think yourself weak,*
> *weak you will be; if you think yourself strong, you will be.*
> —SWAMI VIVEKANANADA, HINDU MONK

## SEVEN DAILY TIPS

For you to thrive, I've broken down what we've covered into seven daily tips. They're in order of importance for you to incorporate one by one:

### 1. Sleep

A great day begins with a good night's sleep. When you're rested, you are more likely to excel in your thinking process, have better cognitive skills, make better choices, including food and beverage choices, exercise, and be in a better mood. There's no compromise. Make your bedroom a sleep sanctuary.

## 2. Movement and Breathing

Physical exercise, movement, postural correction, breathwork, and meditation are all part of how your body moves and breathes. We were not meant to sit at desks all day, and poor posture can inhibit your ability to breathe. Breathing is the most important part of movement and any exercise program.

## 3. Sustenance—Food and Beverages

When it comes to food follow Michael Pollans's three simple rules: eat real food, mostly plants and not too much. When it comes to hydration, upon rising, drink two to three glasses of water. Water is best for the body. Through the day, drink mostly water, consuming little to no other beverages, like soft drinks, coffee or alcohol.

## 4. Love

Love yourself: know you are magnificent and made from divine energy. Connect with people. Be present. Love others. Always, always, always be kind. As George Sand said, "There is only one happiness in this life, to love and be loved."

## 5. Intellect and Intuition

Let curiosity be your guide to find your interests and passions. As humans, we have the ability to transcend time and think about our pasts and our futures. Give your brain the space to breathe, dream, and put forth the vision of what your future looks like. If you think it and work towards it, it has a higher chance to come to be. Success doesn't just find you—you have to go get it.

## 6. Restoration

We need stillness to decompress the mind. Solitude, time alone and time away to think. Creating art, being in nature, or letting the brain wander will give us the respite our spirit needs.

## 7. Dream it. Dream bigger. Dream on.

*When you arise in the morning, think of what*
*a precious privilege it is to be alive— to*
*breathe, to think, to enjoy, to love.*
—MARCUS AURELIUS

# ACKNOWLEDGMENTS

Looking into the abyss of a blank computer screen is terrifying. Then knowing you need to dive head-first into the darkness to find the treasure is even more terrifying. Where does one begin to tell the world about the village it takes to scatter a mountain of words on pages and call it a book?

I have to give a special thanks to my friend and mentor, Elaine Wilkes. She inspired me to dive in and write, that I had a story to tell, and to sit down, and just do it. Then she had the guts to tell me when I needed to do more, to approach my thoughts differently, pushing me to want to scream in frustration—but then I sat down, and dug deeper. Nothing gets by her keen eye for going the distance. I owe her a lot.

The world is a wonderful place. The Internet, books, libraries, documentaries and a deep sense of curiosity can take you wherever you want. There are so many fascinating, smart people in the world doing amazing research and I am eternally grateful they share it on YouTube, TED talks, write books, do documentaries, and push it out into the world for regular people like me to gobble it up. I've done nothing but ask questions and be an observer of other's hard work. I am grateful to everyone.

**Design, Production, Editing, and Illustration Credits**

Content editor: Elaine Wilkes at elaine@elainewilkes.com

Line editors: Ruth Wilkes, Christina Roth and Diane Stockwell, Rachel McClard and Lisa Shartin

Other contributors: Venus Lau and Tony Kurkowski

Cover back photo: Nicole Bisek

Illustrations: Pg55, 52: solar22/Shutterstock.com, Pg66: solar22/iStock.com

Cover graphic image: Dimitrii Guzhanin/Shutterstock.com

Cover design and book layout: Dania Zafar

# ABOUT THE AUTHOR

Past life experiences include biology and respiratory medicine, real estate pension advisory (twice named one of the one hundred most influential people in real estate by *Los Angeles Business Journal*), philanthropist (cofounder of the Boys & Girls Club of Mar Vista Gardens) organ donor, organ recipient, certified instructor in Animal Flow and yoga. Cindy enjoys hobbies that include surfing, doodle drawing, photography, graphic design, writing, teaching, and making barbecue sauce. And now, thanks to all of you she can add published author.

Cindy is married to Jack Jones. Their family include: Jennifer and her husband Joey; John and his wife, Tara; and their kids, Sophia, Trevor, and Henry.

## PHILANTHROPY
**Boys & Girls Club of Mar Vista Gardens**
**Jack and Cindy Jones Youth Center**

Serving over 600 kids with over 140 attending daily housed in the beautifully renovated, 9,000-square-foot facility. To donate, take a tour of the facility, or learn how you can be of service, please visit the website at **www.smbgc.org. (**Boys & Girls Clubs of Santa Monica—Mar Vista Gardens Branch)

## LET'S STAY CONNECTED
🄵 🄾 @Cindy Leuty Jones
🌐 www.gocindyjones.com

# NOTES

1 Dr. Joel Hoomans, "35,000 Decisions: The Great Choices of Strategic Leaders," *Leading Edge Journal*, March 20, 2015, https://go.roberts.edu/leadingedge/the-great-choices-of-strategic-leaders

2 Dara Torres, the twelve-time Olympic medalist, competed in 1984, 1988, 1992, 2000, and 2008 Olympics. In the 2008 Olympics, she won three silver medals in the 4x100 medley relay, 4x100 meter freestyle relay, and 50-meter freestyle. She set a new American record time of 24.07 seconds for the 50-meter freestyle, one one-hundredth (0.01) of a second behind the winner, Britta Steffan. You can't even blink in one one-hundredth of a second.

3 David Rock, "New Study Shows Humans Are on Autopilot Nearly Half the Time," *Psychology Today*, November 14, 2010, https://www.psychologytoday.com/us/blog/your-brain-work/201011/new-study-shows-humans-are-autopilot-nearly-half-the-time

4 National Institute for the Clinical Application of Behavioral Medicine, "Mindless Eating—Would You Notice If Your Popcorn Was Stale?", https://www.nicabm.com/mindless-eating-would-you-notice-if-your-popcorn-was-stale/

5 Saul McLeod, "Maslow's Hierarchy of Needs," *Simply Psychology*, updated 2018, https://www.simplypsychology.org/maslow.html

6 Steven Reiss, "New Theory of Motivation Lists 16 Desires That Guide Us," Ohio State University, June 2000

7 Texas Exes, "University of Texas at Austin 2014 Commencement Address - Admiral William H. McRaven." YouTube, posted May 19, 2014, https://www.youtube.com/watch?v=pxBQLFLei70

8 "Watershed Moment," Grammarist, https://grammarist.com/idiom/watershed-moment/

9 Sarah Knapton, "Deep Breathing Calms You Down Because Brain Cells Spy on Your Breath," *The Telegraph*, March 30, 2017, https://www.telegraph.co.uk/science/2017/03/30/deep-breathing-calms-brain-cell-spy-breath/

10 Mirror Now Digital, "Seven of Ten Most Polluted Cities of the World in 2018 Are in India: Greenpeace Report," Mirrornownews.com, March 06, 2019, https://www.timesnownews.com/mirror-now/in-focus/article/greenpeace-iqair-airvisual-2018-world-air-quality-report-india-gurugram-gurgaon-ghaziabad-faridabad-bhiwadi-noida-patna-lucknow-pollution/377497

11 Ryan Fiorenzi, "Sitting is the New Smoking," Start Standing, July 7, 2019, https://www.startstanding.org/sitting-new-smoking/

12 National Institute of Neurological Disorders and Stroke, "Low Back Pain Fact Sheet," https://www.ninds.nih.gov/Disorders/Patient-Caregiver-Education/Fact-Sheets/Low-Back-Pain-Fact-Sheet

13  Stig Severinsen, "Nitrogen Oxide—A Pleasant Poison!" Breatheology, April 1, 2019, https://www.breatheology.com/nitrogen-oxide-pleasant-poison/

14  Jared Callahan, "Is Breath the Key to Average Joe and Jane Unlocking Their High-Performance Selves?" TheInertia.com, October 25, 2018, https://www.theinertia.com/health/is-breath-the-key-to-average-joe-and-jane-unlocking-their-high-performance-selves/

15  Carl Bialik, "How Much Water Goes into a Burger? Studies Find Different Answers," *Wall Street Journal*, January 11, 2008, https://www.wsj.com/articles/SB120001666638282817

16  Edward McKinley, "Well, Well. The Tap Water in This Kansas City—Area Town Rates among Best in the World," *The Kansas City Star*, August 16, 2019, https://www.kansascity.com/news/local/article233659217.html

17  Christopher S.D. Almond, M.D. et al, "Hyponatremia among Runners in the Boston Marathon," *New England Journal of Medicine*, April 14, 2005, https://www.nejm.org/doi/full/10.1056/nejmoa043901

18  Kathleen M. Zelman, "The Wonders of Water," WebMD Archives

19  Scottie Andrew, "About 40 Percent of American Drink too Much, Study Says," *Newsweek*, July, 7, 2018. https://www.newsweek.com/study-40-percent-americans-drink-too-much-1029294

20  Christopher Ingraham, "Think You Drink a Lot? This Chart Will Tell You." Washington Post, September 25, 2014.

21  A. Bravo et al., "Ingestion of Lactobacillus Strain Regulates Emotional Behavior and Central GABA Receptor Expression in a Mouse via the Vagus Nerve," *Proceedings of the National Academy of Sciences of the United States of America*, September 20, 2011, https://www.ncbi.nlm.nih.gov/pubmed/21876150

22  Diane Nelson, "Breast Milk Reveals Clues for Health," UC Davis New, July 25, 2014, https://www.ucdavis.edu/news/breast-milk-reveals-clues-health/.

23  Ruairi Robertson, "The Gut Microbiome May Affect Your Weight," Healthline, June 27, 2017, https://www.healthline.com/nutrition/gut-microbiome-and-health#section3

24  Akshat Rathi, "Can't lose weight? You Might Be Able to Blame it on Your Parents—And Their Gut Bacteria," Quartz, September 28, 2016, https://qz.com/791056/twins-study-links-gut-bacteria-to-body-fat//

25  "The Microbiome and Weight Gain: Everything We Know So Far," Viome, March 4, 2019, https://www.viome.com/blog/microbiome-and-weight-gain-everything-we-know-so-far

26  "Fibromyalgia Linked to Gut Bacteria for First Time," Technology Networks, June 25, 2019, https://www.technologynetworks.com/neuroscience/news/fibromyalgia-linked-to-gut-bacteria-for-first-time-321033

27  Andrew Siegel, *Finding Your Own Fountain of Youth: The Essential Guide to Maximizing Health, Wellness, Fitness, and Longevity*, (Paul Mould Publishing, 2008) p. 191

28 "Jack LaLanne -LaLanneisms." JackLaLanne.com. archived from the original on February 16, 2010.

29 James Roland, "What's the Average Weight for Men?," *Healthline*, n.d., https://www.healthline.com/health/mens-health/average-weight-for-men

30 Christopher J.L. Murray, Ali Mokdad, and Marie Ng, "The Vast Majority of American Adults Are Overweight or Obese, and Weight is a Growing Problem Among US Children," Healthdata.org, May 28, 2014, http://www.healthdata.org/news-release/vast-majority-american-adults-are-overweight-or-obese-and-weight-growing-problem-among

31 Centers for Disease Control and Prevention, "Long Term Trends in Diabetes," April 2017, https://www.cdc.gov/diabetes/statistics/slides/long_term_trends.pdf

32 Centers for Disease Control and Prevention, "New CDC Report: More Than 100 Million Americans Have Diabetes or Prediabetes," July 18, 2017, https://www.cdc.gov/media/releases/2017/p0718-diabetes-report.html

33 Marlene Busko, "Lifetime Cost of Treating Diabetes in US: Around $85,000," *Medscape*, August 16, 2013, https://www.medscape.com/viewarticle/809547

34 Sean Braswell, "President Eisenhower's $14 Billion Heart Attack," OZY, April 13, 2016, https://www.ozy.com/flashback/president-eisenhowers-14-billion-heart-attack/65157

35 *Sugar Coated*. Directed by Michèle Hozier. 2015. Roxana Spicer, Janice Dawe. Netflix.

36 Healthy Food America, "Sugar Advocacy Tookit, Overview" n.d., http://www.healthyfoodamerica.org/sugartoolkit_overview

37 John Yudkin," Wikipedia, last modified December 6, 2019, https://en.wikipedia.org/wiki/John_Yudkin

38 Joanne Slavin, "Fiber and Prebiotics: Mechanisms and Health Benefits," *MDPI*, April 22, 2013, https://www.ncbi.nlm.nih.gov/pmc/articles/PMC3705355/

39 Riley Cardoza, "Why You Should Be Worried About the Chemicals In Your Hamburger," *Eat This, Not That!*, June 26, 2017, https://www.eatthis.com/hamburger-chemicals/

40 *The Game Changer*, Directed by Louis Psihoyos. 2020. James Cameron, Arnold Schwarzenegger, Jackie Chan, Lewis Hamilton, Novak Djokovic and Chris Paul.

41 Sandra Lösch et al, "Anthropology Unlocks Clues about Roman Gladiators' Eating Habits," Phys.org, October 20th, 2014, https://phys.org/news/2014-10-anthropology-clues-roman-gladiators-habits.html

42 Ibid., *The Game Changer*,

43 M. Wesley Milks, "A Cardiologist's Diet Built for Improving Cholesterol," Medpage Today, October 29, 2019. https://www.medpagetoday.com/cardiology/dyslipidemia/83011

44 Thin Lei Win, "Fighting Global Warming, One Cow Belch At a Time,"

*Reuters*, July 2018, https://www.reuters.com/article/us-global-livestock-emissions/fighting-global-warming-one-cow-belch-at-a-time-idUSKBN1K91CU

45  Brian Palmer, "Can You Die From Lack of Sleep?" *Explainer (blog)*, May 11, 2009, https://slate.com/news-and-politics/2009/05/can-you-die-from-lack-of-sleep.html

46  Danielle Kosecki, "REM, Light, Deep: How Much of Each Stage of Sleep Are You Getting?," Fitbit (blog), September 19, 2018, https://blog.fitbit.com/sleep-stages-explained/

47  Jaclyn Trop, "Drowsy Driving: Worse Than Drunk Driving?" *U.S. News*, December 15, 2016, https://cars.usnews.com/cars-trucks/best-cars-blog/2016/12/drowsy-driving-worse-than-drunk-driving

48  Creative People Remember More Dreams," WebMD, June 27, 2003, https://www.webmd.com/balance/news/20030627/creative-people-remember-more-dreams

49  Megan Wild, "Why a TV Does NOT Belong in the Bedroom," Meet Mindful, n.d., https://www.meetmindful.com/tv-does-not-belong-in-the-bedroom/#

50  Baby Boom," Wikipedia, last modified December 2, 2019, https://en.wikipedia.org/wiki/Baby_boom

51  Kirsten M. J. Thompson, "A Brief History of Birth Control in the U.S.," Our Bodies Ourselves, December 14, 2013, https://www.ourbodiesourselves.org/book-excerpts/health-article/a-brief-history-of-birth-control/

52  "At What Age Is the Brain Fully Developed?" Mental Health Daily, February 18, 2015, https://mentalhealthdaily.com/2015/02/18/at-what-age-is-the-brain-fully-developed/

53  "Abortion Statistics in the United States," Wikipedia, last modified January 2, 2020, https://en.wikipedia.org/wiki/Abortion_statistics_in_the_United_States

54  Prevalence of Birth Control, Wikipedia last modified September 28, 2019, https://en.wikipedia.org/wiki/Prevalence_of_birth_control#cite_note-Hopkins2010-6

55  "8 Things You Probably Didn't Know about Deodorant," Huffington Post, October 15, 2013, https://www.huffpost.com/entry/deodorant-facts_n_4032353

56  Vanessa Marin, "The Difference between Spontaneous and Responsive Desire," Lifehacker.com, September 24, 2018, https://lifehacker.com/the-difference-between-spontaneous-and-responsive-desir-1828754371

57  Emily Nagoski, "How Couples Can Sustain a Strong Sexual Connection for a Lifetime," May 2019, TED Talk video, 9:50, https://www.ted.com/talks/emily_nagoski_how_couples_can_sustain_a_strong_sexual_connection_for_a_lifetime?utm_source=newsletter_weekly_2019-09-27&utm_campaign=newsletter_weekly&utm_medium=email&utm_content=talk_of_the_week_button#t-580870

58  "Rat Park," Wikipedia, https://en.wikipedia.org/wiki/Rat_Park

59  Andreas Komninos, "Safety: Maslow's Hierarchy of Needs," *Interaction Design Foundation*, 2018,

https://www.interaction-design.org/literature/article/safety-maslow-s-hierarchy-of-needs

60  Anxiety and Depression Association of America, "Facts and Statistics," n.d., https://adaa. org/about-adaa/press-room/facts-statistics

61  Jason G. Goldman, "Scientist Reveals Why Great White Sharks Are Targeting California's Shallow Waters," *Los Angeles Magazine*, November 13, 2017, https://www.lamag.com/ mag-features/why-great-white-sharks-targeting-california/

62  Safer America, "2018 Fatal Car Crash Statistics in the U.S.A.," June 27, 2018, https://safer-america.com/2018-fatal-car-crash-statistics-in-the-u-s-a/

63  Bruce Schneier, "Perceived Risk vs. Actual Risk," Schneier.com (blog), November 3, 2006, https://www.schneier.com/blog/archives/2006/11/perceived_risk_2.html

64  Elaina Zachos, "Why Are We Afraid of Sharks? There's a Scientific Explanation," *National Geographic*, June 27, 2019, https://www.nationalgeographic.com/news/2018/01/ sharks-attack-fear-science-psychology-spd/

65  David Rock, "A Hunger for Certainty," *Psychology Today*, October 25, 2009, https://www. psychologytoday.com/us/blog/your-brain-work/200910/hunger-certainty

66  "Dorsolateral Prefrontal Cortex," Wikipedia, last modified December 6, 2019, https://en.wikipedia.org/wiki/Dorsolateral_prefrontal_cortex

67  Denise Grady, "The Vision Thing: Mainly in the Brain," *Discover*, May 31, 1993, http://discovermagazine.com/1993/jun/thevisionthingma227

68  Karin Evans, "Why Forest Bathing Is Good for Your Health," Mindful.org, September 10, 2018, https://www.mindful.org/why-forest-bathing-is-good-for-your-health/

69  "Leonardo di Vinci," Anthony Janson, *History of Art*, 6th ed. (New York: Abrams Books, 2001), 613.

70  Alex Player, "How Marlboro, Coke, and KFC Used Subliminal Advertising," Campaign, February 19, 2016, https://www.campaignlive.co.uk/article/ marlboro-coke-kfc-used-subliminal-advertising/1383489

71  Christopher Bergland, "Subliminal Messages Can Fortify Inner Strength, *Psychology Today*, April 20, 2015, https://www.psychologytoday.com/us/blog/the-athletes-way/201504/ subliminal-messages-can-fortify-inner-strength

72  PCI Global, "Clean Water Is a Human Right," n.d., https://www.pciglobal.org/clean-water/

73  Centers for Disease Control and Prevention, "Diarrhea: Common Illness, Global Killer," n.d., https://www.cdc.gov/healthywater/pdf/global/programs/Globaldiarrhea508c.pdf

74  *Inside Bill's Brain: Decoding Bill Gates*. Directed by Davis Guggenheim. 2019. Alex Bueermann and  Davin Orness. Netflix.

75  Bill Gates, "Why the World Deserves a Better Toilet," Gates Notes, November 5, 2018, https://

www.gatesnotes.com/Development/Sanitation-showcase

76  Abby Norman, "Understanding the Messy, Unreliable Science of Happiness," ATI (All That's Interesting), March 21, 2016, https://allthatsinteresting.com/science-of-happiness

77  "Stanford Marshmallow Experiment," Wikipedia, last modified December 22, 2019, https://en.wikipedia.org/wiki/Stanford_marshmallow_experiment

78  "The Elephant and the Rider," Creative Huddle, April 1, 2016, https://www.creativehuddle.co.uk/the-elephant-and-the-rider

79  Cifford N. Lazarus, "Does Consciousness Exist Outside of the Brain?", Psychology Today (blog), June 26, 2019, https://www.psychologytoday.com/us/blog/think-well/201906/does-consciousness-exist-outside-the-brain

80  Tim Adams, John Cacioppo: 'Loneliness Is Like An Iceberg—It Goes Deeper Than We Can See', *The Guardian*. https://www.theguardian.com/science/2016/feb/28/loneliness-is-like-an-iceberg-john-cacioppo-social-neuroscience-interview

81  Veronique de Turenne, "The Pain of Chronic Loneliness Can Be Detrimental to Your Health." *UCLA Newsroom*, December 2016, https://newsroom.ucla.edu/stories/stories-20161206

82  James E. Dalen et al., "The Epidemic of the 20th Century: Coronary Heart Disease," *The American Journal of Medicine*, May 5, 2014, https://www.amjmed.com/article/S0002-9343(14)00354-4/pdf

83  Ron Grossman and Charles Leroux, "A New 'Roseto Effect,'" *Chicago Tribune*, October 11, 1996, https://www.chicagotribune.com/news/ct-xpm-1996-10-11-9610110254-story.html.

84  Nancy Hayward, "Susan B. Anthony," National Women's History Museum, edited 2018, https://www.womenshistory.org/education-resources/biographies/susan-b-anthony

85  "Chris Kyle," Wikipedia, last modified January 9, 2020, https://en.wikipedia.org/wiki/Chris_Kyle

86  Adam Taylor, "Iraqi Sniper: The Legendary Insurgent Who Claimed to Have Killed Scores of American Troops," *Washington Post*, January 22, 2015 https://www.washingtonpost.com/news/worldviews/wp/2015/01/22/iraqi-sniper-the-legendary-insurgent-who-claimed-to-have-killed-scores-of-american-soldiers/

87  "Keith Richards," Wikipedia, last modified January 9, 2020 https://en.wikipedia.org/wiki/Keith_Richards

88  "Will Rogers," Wikipedia, last modified January 10, 2020, https://en.wikipedia.org/wiki/Will_Rogers

89  Robert Pearl, "The Science of Regrettable Decisions," Vox, July 23, 2019, https://www.vox.com/2019/7/23/20702987/brain-psychology-making-hard-decisions

90  Saul McLeod, "Solomon Asch—Conformity Experiment," *Simply Psychology*, December 28, 2018, https://www.simplypsychology.org/asch-conformity.html

91  Ibid.,

92  Tia Ghose, "Everyone Thinks They Are Above Average," CBS News, February 7, 2013, https://www.cbsnews.com/news/everyone-thinks-they-are-above-average/.

93  James Clear, "Procrastination: A Scientific Guide on How to Stop Procrastinating," JamesClear.com, https://jamesclear.com/procrastination#Why%20Do%20We%20Procrastinate?

94  Carlo Cipolla, last modified January 15, 2020, https://en.wikipedia.org/wiki/Carlo_M._Cipolla: Carlo M. Cipolla, "The Basic Laws of Human Stupidity," n.d., https://web.archive.org/web/20130216132858/http://www.cantrip.org/stupidity.html

95  Carlo M. Cipolla, "The Basic Laws of Human Stupidity," Cantrip.org, n.d., https://www.independent.co.uk/life-style/5-habits-of-stupid-people-that-smart-people-don-t-have-a7620941.html

96  *Inside Bill's Brain: Decoding Bill Gates.* Directed by Davis Guggenheim. 2019. Alex Bueermann and  Davin Orness. Netflix.

97  Thai Nguyen, "10 Proven Ways to Grow Your Brain: Neurogenesis and Neuroplasticity," *Huffington Post*, June 9, 2016, https://www.huffpost.com/entry/10-proven-ways-to-grow-yo_b_10374730

98  Wikipedia, "Hermann Ebbinghaus," https://en.wikipedia.org/wiki/Hermann_Ebbinghaus

99  Robert Mauer, "One Small Step Can Change Your Life," Workman Publishing, New York,

100  Navarro College Cheer Team,  https://navarrocollege.edu/cheer/

101  *Cheer*, Directed by Greg Whiteley. 2020. Boardwalk Pictures, Caviar, One Potato Production. Netflix.

102  Amir Afianian, "What Separates Elite Achievers from Average Performers? A Surprising Finding from the Research behind the So-Called '10,000 hour rule,'" Forge, October 11, 2019, https://forge.medium.com/what-separates-elite-performers-from-the-average-the-berlin-study-c1d00698c030

103  Wikipedia, "*Blink: The Power of Thinking Without Thinking*." https://en.wikipedia.org/wiki/Blink:_The_Power_of_Thinking_Without_Thinking

104  Cari Nierenberg, "The Science of Intuition: How to Measure 'Hunches' and 'Gut' Feelings," Live Science, May 20, 2016, https://www.livescience.com/54825-scientists-measure-intuition.html

105  Eric Barker, "This Is How to Be Your Best Self: 3 Secrets Backed by Research," Bakadesuyo.com, n.d., https://www.bakadesuyo.com/2018/02/best-self/

106  Guy Winch, "Why We Need to Practice Emotional First Aid," November 2014. TED Talk video, 17:15., https://www.ted.com/talks/guy_winch_the_case_for_emotional_hygiene#t-539980

107  "Henri Cartier-Bresson," Wikipedia, https://en.wikipedia.org/wiki/Henri_Cartier-Bresson